Fat Economics

Fat Economics

Nutrition, Health, and Economic Policy

Mario Mazzocchi, W. Bruce Traill, and Jason F. Shogren

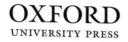

OXFORD

UNIVERSITY PRESS

OXFORD

UNIVERSITY PRESS

Great Clarendon Street, Oxford OX2 6DP

Oxford University Press is a department of the University of Oxford.
It furthers the University's objective of excellence in research, scholarship,
and education by publishing worldwide in

Oxford New York

Auckland Cape Town Dar es Salaam Hong Kong Karachi
Kuala Lumpur Madrid Melbourne Mexico City Nairobi
New Delhi Shanghai Taipei Toronto

With offices in

Argentina Austria Brazil Chile Czech Republic France Greece
Guatemala Hungary Italy Japan Poland Portugal Singapore
South Korea Switzerland Thailand Turkey Ukraine Vietnam

Oxford is a registered trade mark of Oxford University Press
in the UK and in certain other countries

Published in the United States
by Oxford University Press Inc., New York

© Mario Mazzocchi, W. Bruce Traill, and Jason F. Shogren 2009

The moral rights of the authors have been asserted
Database right Oxford University Press (maker)

First published 2009

British Library Cataloguing in Publication Data

Data available

Library of Congress Cataloging in Publication Data

Library of Congress Control Number: 2008942634

Typeset by SPI Publisher Services, Pondicherry, India
Printed in Great Britain
on acid-free paper by
CPI Antony Rowe, Chippenham, Wiltshire

ISBN 978–0–19–921385–6 (hbk.)
      978–0–19–921386–3 (pbk.)

1 3 5 7 9 10 8 6 4 2

To Rafael Carlo, and to Carlo and Mariella
M.M.

To Kathleen, Tom, and Tamsin
W.B.T.

To my family and friends
J.F.S.

Acknowledgements

Many people helped us, knowingly or unknowingly, in the making of this book. We are especially grateful to the many colleagues who gave their insights and remarks on the complex issues dealt with in this book. These include the valuable comments by two anonymous reviewers who read the first draft. Mario Mazzocchi and Bruce Traill wish to thank Bhavani Shankar, Josef Schmidhuber, and Jelle Bruinsma for the stimulating discussions in Reading and Rome, and Elisa Sandri for her help on data processing. Jason Shogren is grateful to Tom Crocker for all the valuable conversations over the years and Linda Thunström for all the discussions on food economics. We are also grateful to the staff of Oxford University Press who helped us through this effort, especially Jennifer Wilkinson, Sarah Caro, and Laurien Berkeley.

As the three authors' institutions are separated by oceans, this book was made possible by the Internet, but also by support from various bodies, including the Institute of Advanced Studies at the University of Bologna, which hosted Bruce Traill in Italy for a fruitful period in 2006. Jason Shogren acknowledges support from Umeå University, Norwegian University of Life Sciences, and GREQAM. Some of the literature and data for this book were collected during Traill and Mazzocchi's previous collaborations with the Food and Agricultural Organization (FAO). However, the contents were written independently of the above collaborations and with no specific funding and FAO is not responsible for any information provided or views expressed.

Contents

List of Figures

List of Tables

List of Tables

Boxes

Abbreviations

BMI	body mass index
BMR	basal metabolic rate
CAP	Common Agricultural Policy (EU)
CARU	Children's Advertising Review Unit (US)
CBA	cost–benefit analysis
CUA	cost–utility analysis
CV	contingent valuation
DALY	disability adjusted life year
DfES	Department for Education and Skills (UK)
FAO	Food and Agriculture Organization
FSA	Food Standards Agency (UK)
GDA	guideline daily amount(s)
GDP	gross domestic product
HDL	high-density lipoprotein
HHP	household production function
IMF	International Monetary Fund
IOTF	International Obesity Task Force
LDL	low-density lipoprotein
LY	life year
NCD	non-communicable disease
NHANES	National Health and Nutrition Examination Survey (US)
NHS	National Health Service (UK)
NICE	National Institute for Health and Clinical Excellence (UK)
NLEA	Nutrition Labeling and Education Act (US)
NSLP	National School Lunch Program (US)
OECD	Organization for Economic Cooperation and Development
QALY	quality adjusted life year
SBP	School Breakfast Program (US)
VAT	value added tax
VSL	value of a statistical life
WHO	World Health Organization
WHR	waist–hip ratio
WTA	willingness-to-accept
WTP	willingness-to-pay

Introduction

For the first time in history overweight people outnumber underweight people.[1] This raises the question whether this is an 'obesity epidemic' and what public policy can or should do about it. Finding tools to understand the question of obesity and unhealthy diets has become a policy priority. In this book, we take an economist's perspective to examine why obesity occurs and what policies might encourage people to make better dietary choices. As has been revealed in other public policy debates (e.g. environment, immigration), economics can explain why some interventions have failed and others succeeded. From an economist's perspective, obesity and health jointly emerge from people's balancing the enjoyment from eating and drinking, and their desire to spend less time in food preparation against the costs of obesity to their health and well-being.

The economic mindset goes beyond basic monetization of costs and benefits or cost-effectiveness studies related to food. The integration of market analysis and behavioral economics into public health is needed for better policy planning. For instance, public health experts distinguish between 'bad nutrition choices' and 'good nutrition choices'. In economics this distinction does not exist. Rather, an economist would address the issue of obesity differently: an informed person chooses to eat a high-calorie diet, avoid physical activity, and become obese because on balance this lifestyle gives him most satisfaction. Information and education, believed to be cure-alls, by themselves do not necessarily solve this problem of bad nutrition choices. A well-informed person may decide to risk

---

[1] The WHO figures actually suggest that there are about 1 billion overweight individuals against 800 million malnourished. This overtaking was communicated by Professor Barry Popkin at the 2006 meeting of the International Association of Agricultural Economists in Brisbane and received large attention by the press; see e.g. 'Overweight People Now Outnumber the Hungry', *The Telegraph*, 16 Aug. 2006; 'Overweight "Top World's Hungry"', BBC News, 15 Aug. 2006, <http://news.bbc.co.uk/1/hi/health/4793455.stm>.

long-term adverse health in favor of short-term gratification. Information is a precondition of good diet choice, but not necessarily the most effective policy for improving diets. When comparing the costs and benefits of their decisions, informed consumers may change their behavior in response to changes in their circumstances, like an increase in their health insurance costs, a change in the price of a 'bad diet' compared to a 'healthy diet', a rise in their incomes, or a reduction in their free time. Economics stresses the importance of exploring such changes facing individuals and using appropriate statistical models to derive a robust evidence base of cause and effect.

In the book, we discuss how the applied economics literature has examined health policy and other relevant areas. We provide a systematic and critical review of the existing evidence. We make no apologies for introducing and applying the tools of economic analysis, as economics has developed a useful toolkit to examine such questions and to assess the social and private costs and benefits and appropriateness of government policies. That said, we recognize that economics does not have all the answers to all questions. For instance, we do not contribute to the scientific debate about diet–health relationships and we accept what nutritionists tell us in this respect. We have little to say on practical questions of how best to establish and operate public health interventions, for example a community-based advice and weight-loss scheme. Also, psychologists, anthropologists, and sociologists have made important contributions to understanding individual and societal behavior.

Rationale of the Book

A person's body weight arises from a multitude of factors, including genetics, social determinants, psychological traits, and economic drivers. We wrote this book because the contribution from the economic community to public health debates on obesity and other diet-related causes of ill health is little understood and underrepresented. We challenge the myth that economics is highbrow theory based on unrealistic assumptions. Rather, we provide a discussion grounded in the real world, using practical examples and a critical assessment of empirical outcomes.

One area in which economics can make a contribution is in the understanding of markets and their sometimes seemingly perverse behavior. Consider two examples that illustrate our approach. First, a consensus exists about the health benefits of raising fruit and vegetable consumption and the '5-a-day' target, which has been supported by information campaigns throughout the world. If all 60 million people in the UK ate the recommended 400 grams of fruit and vegetables per day, the total demand would increase to about 9 million tons per year from 2005 consumption of about 7 million tons. Food and Agriculture Organization figures show that domestic production in 2005 was around 3 million tons.[2] It would be obviously impossible for domestic production to expand sufficiently to supply the increased demand; this would require a near doubling of output. The additional demand would have to be met mainly through imports, which would result in a likely increase in prices.

The extent of the price rise is the key to the success or failure of the 5-a-day campaign and depends on many interrelated factors: How much and how quickly would domestic production respond? How much would prices rise in the short and long terms? Would higher prices offset the increased demand to a noticeable extent (how much do consumers react to price changes)? These are the sorts of issues empirical economics addresses, and policy decisions that do not recognize existing market conditions and potential consumer response may lead to unexpected, possibly adverse, outcomes, especially in the short term. The policymaker should recognize that the information effect may be less successful than anticipated if greater demand results in increased prices which in turn reduce demand for fruit and vegetables.

Another market-related example we explore is how agricultural policies affect diets. Some observers claim that Europe's Common Agricultural Policy (CAP) contributes to the obesity epidemic because it subsidizes farmers, especially those producing unhealthy sugar, butter, and cream. Subsidization of sugar and milk results in increased production, and, they argue, more consumption. The CAP does subsidize farmers, especially sugar and dairy producers, but it does so by intervening in markets to raise prices to consumers and producers. How do producers react to rising prices? They produce more. How do consumers react to rising prices? They consume less—and switch to lower-priced alternatives. The main impact of the CAP is to reduce consumption of products whose prices rise

---

[2] These figures are based on data on per capita consumption from the UK Department for Environment, Food, and Rural Affairs (<http://www.defra.gov.uk>), which estimates fruit and vegetable consumption at about 320 grams per capita per day in 2005 and on production data from FAOSTAT (<http://www.fao.org>), which estimates production of fruit and vegetables at 3.1 million tons for the same year.

most, sugar and dairy products, and encourage consumption of foods whose prices do not increase (or not as much), such as healthy fruit and vegetables.[3] CAP subsidies are good for our diets! To address the question of how it is possible that more is produced but less is consumed, think back to 'butter mountains' and 'wine lakes', and recognize that smaller amounts of sugar and dairy products are imported and larger quantities are exported than would be the case in Europe without the CAP.

Economists also take a broader perspective on public policy toward health. Economists view health policy as a two-way street: income affects health and health affects income. People make choices and a feedback is created between our ability to accrue wealth and maintain health. While this mindset seems straightforward enough, it has a deeper implication. Economics plays a larger role in public health policy than previously acknowledged. Economic circumstances (e.g. prices, incomes) help to determine what we choose to eat, how much we eat, whether we exercise a lot or a little, and what priority we give to preventive medical care. We are not driven by biology and physiology alone; rather, these interact with human behavior to determine health and other outcomes. Among other implications, this suggests that economics should be an integrated element within public health policy, not just an afterthought to determine whether policy is cost-effective. In other words, human behavioral response should be considered at the outset, during policy formulation. It should be recognized that health and welfare are jointly determined by economic and biological circumstances.

Why? Human behavior and private decision making underpin public policy toward diet and health. The logic works as follows: people make food and exercise decisions based on health status, preferences, location, and so on; economic circumstances affect these private decisions because the prices of different foods and our incomes and wealth affect the quantity and quality of food we buy. Any policy aimed at changing how people eat has to account for how these economic variables might change and how people will adapt to that change—by altering either their food purchases or their exercise regime. Economists believe that diet and health policy can be improved by integrating these economic circumstances into the core of the biomedical and public health disciplines. Understanding the driving forces affecting people's decisions and understanding the feedback between these choices and health is crucial for better policy. To achieve this it is necessary to go beyond a 'natural science, first; then economics' approach that merely adds a set of medical parameters

---

[3] Ritson (1998).

into economic models or vice versa. A central message of this book is that economics matters to health policy at the most fundamental level.

These ideas go beyond conceptual issues. Critical empirical issues arise, and economists have developed models that move beyond epidemiological relationships which neglect adaptation in human behavior. For example, an epidemiological model might estimate a relationship between salt intake and blood pressure holding all other variables constant and observe that higher salt intake is associated with higher blood pressure. The prescription would be to reduce population salt intake. By contrast an economic model would recognize that all other variables do not remain constant; if people find that salt makes vegetables more palatable, when reducing their salt intake they might also reduce vegetable consumption, which in turn may lead to adverse health outcomes including higher blood pressure.[4] An empirical economic model therefore allows other variables in the model to readjust to reflect actual consumer behavior.

Take another, more intuitive, piece of research from outside the nutrition literature, but still referring to health and risk adjustment. The public health literature has looked at the relationship between fire deaths in homes in the US and the presence of fire detectors; they find that a 1% increase in fire detectors in homes reduces deaths by 0.46% when holding all other variables constant (people's incomes, other fire safety devices, etc.). By contrast, an economic model incorporates income into the relationship and finds that a 1% increase in fire detectors in homes only reduces deaths by 0.1%.[5] Why the discrepancy? The economic model recognizes that richer people are not only more likely to install fire detectors but also purchase other fire safety equipment, choose to live in safer locations, and are less likely to smoke. The difference in the magnitude of the effects between economic and public health models is because the public health model attributes all the factors associated with safer houses and lifestyles to fire detectors. Properly accounted for, it turns out that while detectors are still effective, they are much less so than had been thought.

Throughout the book we use such real-world examples to illustrate the insight gained from adopting the economist's perspective in obesity policy.

---

[4] The change in sign of the relationship between salt intake and blood pressure when moving from an epidemiological to economic model is an actual empirical finding in Chen et al. (2002).

[5] Garbacz and Thompson (2007).

Intended Audience

This book is targeted at professionals in the health care sector with an interest or responsibility in health and nutrition interventions, who may benefit from a better understanding of the potential and limits of the economic approach. This includes researchers in the public health sector and health economists, who are likely to be aware of the role of economics, and might appreciate a thorough review of the literature and the focus on the empirical successes and failures of economics in explaining obesity and other diet-related adverse outcomes.

Structure of the Book

The book begins with a description of the so-called 'obesity epidemic'. Chapter 1 provides a closer look at the numbers behind the epidemic. We go beyond the statistics and economic figures which fill the introductions of most books and articles. For example, Philipson (2001) points out that the shape of the distribution of body mass index (BMI) as well as the mean are important; obesity rates can go up even when median population weight is unchanged if there is weight gain in the right-hand tail of the BMI distribution (i.e. if those who are already overweight become obese while normal-weight people's weight doesn't change). This would be important in determining whether policy interventions should be targeted at the population or a subgroup. For example, suppose a government aims to reach the World Health Organization 'population' target of 400 grams of fruit and vegetables per capita per day. Assuming a symmetric distribution of fruit and vegetable consumption among the population, achieving the target 'on average' means that half of the population is below the target. Is this the intention of the intervention? 5-a-day campaigns seem to suggest that everyone should consume five 80 gram portions per day, but given that some people consume more, this implies that the average for the population should be above 400 grams. This is an important distinction when it comes to evaluation of policy effectiveness.

Chapter 2 moves onto the fundamental question: what motivates people to eat more than they should or choose bad diets? Here the challenge is to navigate the literature. With the help of economics we extend the search for the real culprits, moving beyond the circle of the usual suspects. For example, most economists now recognize that technological change is a key factor, since it acts in both directions on the calorie equation: technology makes it easier, cheaper, and more convenient to get calories, through microwaves and ready meals, but also makes it more difficult to spend calories, with cars, computers, and cable television. But some key factors are less obvious. According to economic decision making, we all 'discount' the future consequences of our current decisions. If the harmful consequences of unhealthy lifestyles are delayed to older age, younger people live for today and place less emphasis on long-term harmful consequences. This might be an alternative or additional explanation for why younger generations eat worse diets than older generations, and also raises questions about the likely effectiveness of nutrition education measures to reduce obesity in young people that emphasize adverse health outcomes. Perhaps they should put greater emphasis on short-term factors like physical attractiveness.

Chapter 3 uses the economic toolkit to quantify the damage. Again, our goal is to illustrate how standard procedures are incomplete. When the economic dimension is added, the assessment of the costs of obesity and the benefits of intervention are less straightforward than one would expect. We distinguish between private costs, payable by the individual as a consequence of his free choices, and the social costs borne by the rest of society. If a person *chooses* to overeat knowing full well the probability of his suffering ill health later in life *and* he will personally bear the full costs resulting from his choices, it cannot be said that there are positive benefits from an intervention to encourage or cajole him to eat more healthily; if, however, the costs of his ill health are borne by society as a whole, it is necessary to measure these costs and benefits in some way. We discuss alternative measures such as quality adjusted life years, and their interpretation and appropriateness in different circumstances. Real-world case studies are used to support the conceptual analysis.

Chapter 4 explores the range of policy measures aimed at reducing obesity and the empirical evidence for their effectiveness. The measures include fiscal policies (taxes and subsidies), information and education campaigns, restrictions on advertising, legal liability, reformulation of foods, and so forth. Some insight can be gained from the experience of smoking policies, although it is important to draw the line between the two public health issues underlining differences as well as similarities.

Chapter 5 summarizes the evidence and identifies remaining questions. What will be the future? How could undesirable actions be prevented rather than punished? And how has the economics perspective helped? Can we get better health at lower costs?

References

Chen, S. N., J. F. Shogren, P. F. Orazem, and T. D. Crocker (2002), 'Prices and Health: Identifying the Effects of Nutrition, Exercise, and Medication Choices on Blood Pressure', *American Journal of Agricultural Economics*, 84/4: 990–1002.

Garbacz, C., and H. G. Thompson (2007), 'Are Smoke Detectors as Effective as the Public Health Literature Reports?', *Economics Letters*, 97/1: 11–16.

Philipson, T. J. (2001), 'The World-Wide Growth in Obesity: An Economic Research Agenda', *Health Economics*, 10/1: 1–7.

Ritson, C. (1998), 'Agenda 2000', *Nutrition and Food Science*, 98/4: 198–201.

1

The Obesity Epidemic

Each day we read and hear more about obesity in the press and on TV. A recent Google search[1] uncovered the following among the multitude of headlines:

'Obesity crisis tops 14m' (in Britain)
'Scottish diet hard-wires kids to be fat'
'Soft drinking teens pile on pounds'
'Couch potato clue to obesity epidemic'
'American food manufacturers may be contributing to the obesity epidemic'
'Food lobby weighs in on obesity debate'
'Obesity on verge of surpassing smoking as #1 cause of preventable death'
'Obesity can lead to blindness'
'Breast cancer link to childhood obesity probed'
'80,000 cancer death cases caused by diet'
'Children falling victim to "adult" diabetes'
'Medical cost of obesity $75b'
'Big spend for obese beds'
'Junk food ads to be banned from kids' TV'
'Too little done to cut obesity'
'The obesity epidemic: why and how the government must act'
'Society must act to cut obesity'
'Industry could help halt rising tide of obesity'.

---

[1] At the time of writing, a Google search for 'obesity epidemic' returned about 1,070,000 hits. Cited titles refer to articles which appeared on *The Sun* online, *The Times*, the *Daily Mail*, *New Scientist*, the International Obesity Task Force Conference web site, BBC News, the American Obesity Association web site, and CNN.com, between 2004 and 2006.

These headlines reveal the current conventional wisdom: people in developed nations are facing an obesity epidemic and the problem is going to get worse, especially given the growing prevalence of childhood obesity; the problem is caused by people eating too much junk food, sugary soft drinks, and processed foods as well as forgoing exercise; obesity has caused a dramatic increase in the prevalence of non-communicable diseases such as diabetes, cancer, hypertension, and heart disease; these obesity-related diseases are imposing huge costs on health systems; government policies are partly to blame for the epidemic and industry also promotes obesity by producing and promoting unhealthy foods, especially targeted at children—they must both do 'something' to remedy the situation, as must 'society'.

Our aim in this book is to look behind the headlines. While some scientists still debate whether the obesity 'epidemic' matters at all,[2] we know that addressing obesity is a priority on the policy agenda. We introduce the issue by looking at the existing figures on obesity, food consumption, exercise, and health so readers less familiar with the subject can gain an overview of the problem. We also highlight questions that arise when looking at less obvious aspects of the data behind the headlines. For example, why is obesity much more prevalent in some countries than others? Is it correct to view obesity and its health consequences as a population problem or as one that affects only segments of society, perhaps definable by age, race, or social class? If the latter, to what extent are the differences behaviorally based rather than biological?[3] And what are the implications for targeted policy interventions? Finally, we introduce the economist's perspective on the obesity challenge and indicate where in the book the various issues are considered in more detail. Again we emphasize that economics does not address all aspects of the problem, and sometimes, for those it does address, the economic approach is hampered by incomplete data. Nevertheless, we argue that the economist's perspective provides insight into the challenges and raises questions overlooked by others.

---

[2] Oliver (2006) provides many counterarguments in that respect.

[3] Among innovative theories on the causes of obesity, some scientists are arguing that the epidemic might be fueled by biological factors, possibly even an obesity virus. These studies stem from empirical observations of 'transmission' of obesity within social networks, which obviously can also be explained by behavioral factors. See Christakis and Fowler (2007); Dhurandhar (2001).

The 'Epidemic' in Context

We begin by looking at international trends in overweight and obesity. We examine the changes in energy intake and expenditure responsible for the gains in weight over the past decades and discuss the health consequences of overweight and obesity.

Obesity and Overweight

The body mass index (BMI) is the most widely used indicator of excess weight and obesity.[4] BMI is defined as weight in kilograms divided by height in meters squared. A person is defined as *overweight* if their BMI is between 25 and 30, *obese* if BMI exceeds 30. Normal weight is defined as the BMI range 18.5 to 25, with BMI below 18.5 being underweight. Many developed countries have just started keeping official records of the proportions of people in overweight and obese categories; many developing countries have just started to be aware of the magnitude of the problem.

Table 1.1 shows overweight and obesity prevalence in the OECD countries. Except for the United States, all countries with data going back to 1980 show low levels of obesity, below 10% of the population. But many countries have seen obesity increase substantially over the past twenty-five years. The US, now joined by Mexico, has the highest rate of obesity—over 30% of the population, with the other Anglo-Saxon countries as well as Greece, Hungary, and Luxembourg with obesity prevalence around 20%. Many countries have obesity rates around 10% of their population, with only Japan and Korea showing rates below 5%.

The proportion of the population which is overweight is between 20% and 30% in almost all countries, with Japan slightly below and the UK and Mexico above. Unlike obesity, there are downward trends in the rate of overweight in some countries as well as upward trends in others.

When the numbers of overweight and obese are combined, Mexico, the United States, and the UK lead the pack with 66%, 61%, and 55% of adults; Norway has 35% and Japan only 20% per cent. The prevalence of overweight and obese individuals is increasing over time in almost all OECD

---

[4] An alternative measure of body weight is the waist–hip ratio (WHR), i.e. the ratio of the circumference of the waist to that of the hips. Recent epidemiological research has shown the failure of BMI in predicting health outcomes, especially cardiovascular diseases, suggesting that WHR is a better predictor of health (Kragelund and Omland 2005). However, there are no internationally comparable figures on WHR.

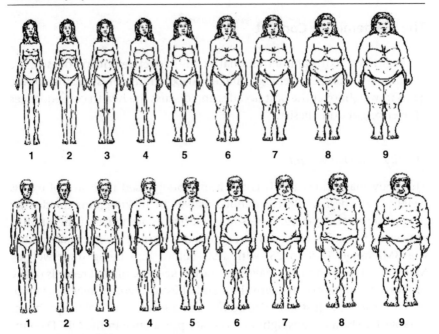

FIG. 1.1. Diagrammatic representation of BMI in women and men

1 = BMI of 16; 2 = BMI of 19; 3 = BMI of 22; 4 = BMI of 25; 5 = BMI of 28; 6 = BMI of 31; 7 = BMI of 34; 8 = BMI of 37; 9 = BMI of 40.

Source: Pulvers et al. (2004).

countries for which there are two or more data points. In general, men tend to be more overweight than women, but the prevalence of obesity is equally likely to be higher among women.

It is unclear from these data how to interpret the disparate trends between overweight and obesity rates. We do not know whether there has been a rightward shift in the entire frequency distribution of weight, with everyone having become somewhat heavier, or if most people's weight is unchanged but a susceptible few have become obese. To assess in more detail what is happening requires more information on the entire frequency distribution, and for this we need to look within countries at individual-level data. We return to this issue in a moment. First, we ask whether we can 'explain' cross-country differences in obesity. Casual observation suggests that this is difficult: the four leaders in the obesity stakes, the US, UK, Mexico, and Greece appear to have little in common. Likewise, a group of European countries show moderately low levels of obesity, around 10%, but they are a disparate group geographically and

12

Table 1.1. Adult overweight and obesity rates in OECD countries, 1980–2005 (% of population with BMI 25–30 and BMI >30)

	Overweight				Obese			
	1980	1990	2000	2005	1980	1990	2000	2005
Australia	18.7	23.8[a]	28.2[b]		8.3	10.8[a]	21.7[b]	
Austria		21.3[b]				8.5[c]	9.1[b]	
Belgium			25.7[d]	24.4[e]			11.7[d]	
Canada		25.1[f]	25.0[d]	24.7		12.1[f]	13.9[d]	18.0
Czech Republic		28.3[g]	30.7[h]	29.0		11.2[g]	14.8[h]	17.0
Denmark			24.9	26.4		5.5[i]	9.5	11.4
Finland	24.2	21.8	25.7	26.6	7.4	8.4	11.2	14.1
France		18.8	20.1	19.6[e]		5.8	9.0	9.5[e]
Germany			28.7[b]	28.7			11.5[b]	13.6
Greece				29.9[j]				21.9[j]
Hungary			28.5	29.8[j]			18.2	18.8[j]
Iceland			28.0				12.4[h]	
Ireland			25.0[h]				13.0[h]	
Italy		24.4[f]	25.1	26.2		7.5[f]	8.6	9.9
Japan	17.9	19.1	18.1	16.9[e]	2.0	2.3	2.9	3.0[e]
Korea, Republic of			25.9[d]	23.7			3.2[d]	3.5
Luxembourg			24.2	25.4			16.3	18.6
Mexico			35.8	36.6			24.2	30.2
Netherlands	23.4[k]	23.7	30.2	28.2	5.1[k]	6.1	9.4	10.7
New Zealand		25.0[a]	30.1[l]	28.4[j]		11.1[a]	17.0[l]	20.9[l]
Norway		20.3[m]	23.2[h]	26.0		5.0[m]	8.3[h]	9.0
Poland			26.5[n]	26.6[e]			11.4[n]	12.5[e]
Portugal			31.8[b]				12.8[b]	
Slovak Republic				24.9[j]		18.9[g]	16.2[o]	15.4[j]
Spain		23.9[i]	27.8[d]	27.6[j]		6.8[i]	12.6[d]	13.1[j]
Sweden			26.6	25.9		5.5[a]	9.2	10.7
Switzerland		17.1[p]	21.8[h]			5.4[p]	7.7[h]	
Turkey				28.9[j]				12.0[j]
United Kingdom	24.0	29.0[c]	33.8	32.1	7.0	14.0[c]	21.0	23.0
United States	25.0[q]	25.3[c]	28.5	28.6	15.0[q]	23.3[c]	30.5	32.2[e]

Note: BMI = body mass index defined as weight in kilograms divided by height in meters squared.

[a] 1989.　　[b] 1999.　　[c] 1991.　　[d] 2001.　　[e] 2004.　　[f] 1994.　　[g] 1993.　　[h] 2002.
[i] 1987.　　[j] 2003.　　[k] 1981.　　[l] 1997.　　[m] 1995.　　[n] 1996.　　[o] 1998.　　[p] 1992.
[q] 1978.

Source: OECD Health Data (2007), <http://oberon.sourceoecd.org>.

culturally, ranging from Norway to Italy (though Germany and Spain are somewhat higher—why?). Two regularities are that the transition economies of east and central Europe have consistently high levels of obesity and the Asian duo of Korea and Japan have low rates.

Several theories have been put forward to explain apparent cross-country sdifferences in obesity, none entirely convincing. Differences may be simply down to different methods of data collection, though in the developed OECD nations, such data should be relatively easy to collect, thus reliable. Assuming the differences are meaningful, one theory is that countries with low levels of 'individualism' and associated high levels of community involvement and regulation (Japan, Korea, Italy, Scandinavia) tend to be less obese than those with high levels of individualism and reliance on the free market, such as the Anglo-Saxon countries.[5] Another is that countries with a strong food tradition (France, Italy, Japan, Korea) have made fewer dietary adjustments, and are less obese, than those which lack a strong food culture.[6] Basic economics suggests that income and price differences affect food choice and urbanization influences energy expenditure, but regressions which use obesity rate as the dependent variable and the price of food, income, measures of culture,[7] and other variables as independent variables explain little of the cross-country variation. A further complication in understanding cross-country differences in obesity rates, as shown later in this chapter, is that recent data on children seem to indicate differing trends from those seen in the adult population, as 'traditionally thin' countries are experiencing rapidly increasing rates of childhood obesity, some higher than those recorded in the US.

The trend toward obesity in the Western world is not a surprise. What is more unexpected is its reach into the developing world. The prevalence of overweight people is already reaching similar proportions in Latin America, the Middle East, and the European transition states as in the developed world, and the numbers overweight have overtaken those underweight in China, several other Asian countries, and even some of the poorest parts of Africa, as shown in Table 1.2, which uses data drawn together by Mendez and Popkin from surveys in a number of middle-income and developing countries.[8] In fact, in September 2006, the World Health Organization (WHO) announced that overweight people now number 1,000 million in the world (300 million obese) compared to 800 million underweight. Developing countries are suffering what has been termed the double burden of malnutrition:[9] the coexistence of overweight and underweight people within a single country and within a single family.

Understanding cross-country differences in obesity has proved difficult. We turn now to the evidence within a country. Accumulating evidence (almost entirely from the US) suggests that the right-hand tail of the BMI frequency distribution has grown, indicating that those susceptible to

---

[5] Cutler et al. (2003); Hofstede (2001).

[6] See e.g. Lang and Heasman (2004).

[7] Hofstede, a psychologist, has 'measured culture across 4 dimensions, individualism, masculinity, power distance and uncertainty avoidance'; see e.g. Hofstede (2001).

[8] Up-to-date figures from surveys in these and other countries can also be accessed through the WHO web site at <http://www.who.int/infobase/report.aspx?rid=112&ind=BMI>.

[9] Schmidhuber and Shetty (2005).

Table 1.2. Over- and underweight proportions of the female population aged 20–49 in the late 1990s (%)

Country	Overweight[a]		Underweight[b]	
	Urban	Rural	Urban	Rural
Latin America				
Bolivia (1998)	57.9	47.1	7.4	6.1
Brazil (1996)	42.8	33.0	5.2	9.3
Colombia (2000)	48.8	51.4	2.0	2.1
Mexico (1999)	65.4	58.6	1.5	2.2
Peru (2000)	60.2	43.3	0.8	0.7
Transition economies				
Kazakhstan (1999)	36.3	36.3	6.3	6.0
Kyrgyzstan (1997)	34.7	34.5	4.9	4.4
Middle East, Eurasia				
Egypt (1995)	69.9	46.6	0.7	1.8
Jordan (1997)	69.4	63.0	1.6	1.8
Turkey (1998)	63.2	65.6	2.1	1.5
South and Southeast Asia				
China (1997)	20.5	15.2	7.4	6.1
India (1999)	26.4	5.6	23.1	48.3

[a] BMI >25.
[b] BMI <18.5.

Source: Mendez and Popkin (2004).

weight gain have put on more weight than the average person: the rise in the proportion of obese people has risen much more sharply than the rise in average weight. Between the 1970s and the 1999–2000 US National Health and Nutrition Examination Survey, as far as we know the only survey in the world repeated over a long enough time to capture the emergence and full development of the obesity epidemic, median BMI among adults increased from 24.6 to 26.3 (or by 8.9%), whereas at the 95% tail of the distribution it rose from 33.9 to 39.6 (or by 16.8%). A similar shift in the shape of the distribution took place for children.[10] This suggests that those people susceptible to obesity (by virtue of their genes, environment, or personality) have become much more obese over time, but the average person has only shown a small weight gain.

English data over a shorter period and not from a single source appear to support this finding. Figure 1.2 illustrates what happened to the BMI distribution in England between 1986 and 2005 compared to US data between 1971 and 2006. According to the individual data, during this period the obesity rate in England jumped from 10% to 25% and the

[10] Anderson et al. (2003).

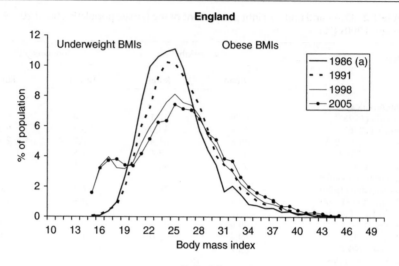

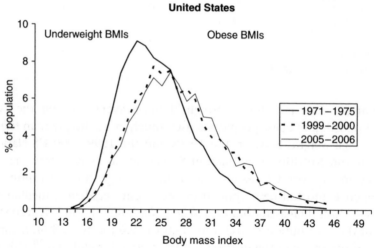

Fɪɢ. 1.2. Evolution of the distribution of body mass index in England (1986–2005) and the United States (1971–2006)

Data for 1986–7 refer to Britain; 1991, 1998, and 2005 to England. All data refer to adults (over 18) only.

Sources: Our processing on data from Dietary and Nutritional Survey of British Adults, 1986–7; Health Survey for England (1991, 1998, 2005); US National Health and Nutrition Examination Survey (1971–5, 1999–2000, 2005–6).

prevalence of obese or overweight individuals increased from 41% to 64%.[11] While the 1986 and 1991 curves show a single peak around the median value, as we move into the 1990s the distribution becomes 'flatter', with bigger tails, and is less regular, with a clear peak in the underweight part of the graph, suggesting the development of other eating disorders. US data on adult BMI show a clear shift of the mean and median value toward the right between 1971 and 2000 (but not between 2000 and 2006), as well as a higher right tail, while the prevalence of underweight individuals declines over time.

These shifts raise a key point: the tendency to gain weight is not a general trend. Policies need to be targeted: placing too much emphasis on eating less for the whole population might be unnecessary for many and could even create an unintended consequence for some who may already be undereating. Thus, it becomes crucial to understand *who* are underweight, overweight, or obese and target policies accordingly.

In developed countries, obesity is recognized as a problem among the lower socio-economic groups and ethnic minorities. This pattern is being replicated in middle-income developing countries. Popkin and Ng (2006) report that for all countries with annual income per capita over $US2,500 (e.g. Thailand, Bulgaria, and Tunisia) the prevalence of obesity among women was inversely related to socio-economic status. Age is the variable most closely associated with weight gain. Analysis of English data[12] indicates that, holding everything else constant, the likelihood of being overweight increases gradually up to the age of 75, by when people are four times as likely to be overweight as at age 16–25. The likelihood of being obese peaks earlier, in the 45–55 age group (when it is about twice as likely as for a 16–25-year-old), then falls somewhat. In England people in the lowest social class (E) are around 25% more likely to be overweight or obese than those in the highest social class (A). The only group in which obesity levels are falling over time is social class A females. The same phenomenon has been observed, over a longer period, in Japan.

Looking to the future, health experts are concerned about the sharp rise in childhood obesity—and the observation that obese children are more

---

[11] Very minor discrepancies from OECD data are due to aggregation weights.

[12] From the Health Survey for England, using logistic regression with overweight/obese as the dependent variable and age, social class, and other demographic variables as independent variables.

likely than thin children to become obese adults. But in making such statements we need to recognize that most obese adults were not overweight as children and not all obese children go on to become obese adults. This implies that when we discuss the economic causes of obesity in subsequent chapters we must examine the forces that cause both adults and children to become obese. The causality of the relationships between child and adult obesity is further complicated by the observation that children are more likely to be overweight or obese if they have overweight or obese parents. The Department of Health has calculated that in England more than 20% of children with two obese or overweight parents are themselves overweight or obese (BMI >25) compared to only 7% when both parents are normal weight,[13] and, for girls, being in an overweight– obese household means a threefold increase in the odds of being obese compared to normal-weight households.[14]

According to the International Obesity Task Force (IOTF),[15] the prevalence of overweight or obese children among English 2–15-year-olds has increased dramatically from 10% in the mid-1980s to 27% in 2002, of which 6% were obese compared to 1% in the 1980s. There are other striking data for overweight and obese children at the beginning of the twenty-first century; official statistics show about 1 child in 3 between the ages of 6 and 13 is overweight or obese in Italy whereas 'only' 1 child in 5 is overweight or obese in the US. Other southern European countries like Greece and Spain show rates similar to Italy, but throughout Europe childhood overweight rates have already reached the US rates.[16] Globally, the IOTF has estimated that 1 in 10 children is overweight or obese, representing 155 million children.[17]

In summary, the data raise as many questions as answers. The one thing all data point to is that the proportion of overweight and obese people has been increasing in virtually all countries. While large differences exist across countries (in prevalence and trends), perhaps the critical fact is that childhood obesity rates are highest in several Mediterranean countries where adult obesity is relatively low. Limited data within countries

---

[13] Data based on the 2001/2002 National Diet and Nutrition Survey, NHS Information Centre, *Statistics on Obesity, Physical Activity and Diet: England, 2006*, <http://www.ic.nhs.uk/webfiles/publications/obesity/StatisticsOnObesity201206_PDF.pdf>.

[14] Data based on the 2006 Health Survey for England, National Statistics and NHS Information Centre, *Statistics on Obesity, Physical Activity and Diet: England, January 2008*, <http://www.ic.nhs.uk/pubs/opadjan08>.

[15] See Cole et al. (2000) for a rigorous definition of child overweight and obesity cut-off points.

[16] Lobstein and Frelut (2003).

[17] <http://www.iotf.org/childhoodobesity.asp>.

suggest that people in most social groups are becoming heavier and greater attention needs to be paid to the right tail of the BMI frequency distribution. Obese people seem to be putting on weight more quickly than the population at large. Age, gender, and social group are all associated with obesity, as is ethnicity, which suggests the need to understand better the forces at work on different groups. 'One size fits all' policy interventions are unlikely to be successful.

The Nutrition Transition

Consider now the underlying biological causes of weight gain over time. People gain weight because their energy intake exceeds their energy output, so an upward trend in weight implies people are eating more calories, getting less exercise, or both. Calories are needed to maintain basic body functions, to digest food, and for exercise. The energy needs of basic body maintenance increase with weight; a simplified expression of the number of calories needed to maintain resting weight (known as the basal metabolic rate, BMR) is expressed as:

$$BMR = a + b^*weight$$

where weight is measured in kilograms. While genetic differences exist in how many calories are needed to perform this function, an average value for a is 879 for men, 829 for women, and b is 11.6 for men and 8.7 women.[18]

About 10% of food energy is used for digestion. Energy is also needed to exercise, with the number of calories used depending on the intensity of the exercise, its duration, and the weight of the person. For example, light work such as housework requires around 3.5 times a person's BMR, gentle walking around 2.3 times BMR.

Combining these three ways of using energy, a person's steady state weight can be calculated by their level of exercise and their intake of calories, or conversely we can calculate their calorie requirement to maintain their present weight. According to this calculation, a genetically average male of say 80 kilograms exercising at a moderate level, so that his average energy requirement per day was twice his BMR, would need

---

[18] See Cutler et al. (2003); Harris and Benedict (1918). The original equation also allowed for variation associated with height and age but we have subsumed these into the intercept at reasonable 'average' levels.

3,038 calories per day to maintain body weight; a woman of 60 kilograms would need 1,887 calories per day.

Looked at another way, if the man consumed an extra 100 calories per day, every day, without modifying his exercise, his steady state weight would increase over time to 83.8 kilograms—a substantial weight gain, 5%, for a small increase in calorie intake (3%, or a can of soft drink per day). Between the 1960s and the early 2000s, calorie availability in developing countries increased from 1,950 to 2,680 calories per capita per day;[19] in the EU-15 it increased from 2,984 calories per capita per day to 3,505 calories per capita per day over the same period.[20]

Energy (or calorie) availability differs from energy (or calorie) intake because it does not account for household waste such as peeling fruit and vegetables, feeding scraps to pets, and throwing away used cooking oil. Availability corresponds more closely to food purchased than food consumed. This implies that both the levels and increases in availability are overestimates of actual consumption and consumption increases. But unless the proportion of food wasted has increased dramatically, the proportionate increase in energy intake is realistic: about 37% in developing countries, 17% in the EU.[21] Table 1.3 shows trends in different world areas over the period 1990–2005. While calorie availability is increasing in most areas (an exception is middle Africa, with the lowest availability level), rates are higher in those countries where an increase in obesity prevalence has been observed.

---

[19] Schmidhuber and Shetty (2005).

[20] Schmidhuber and Traill (2006).

[21] We include a warning with this statement: some developed countries have been calculating energy intake from detailed surveys of household food consumption for many years. These are considered by nutritionists to be the gold standard as regards food consumption data, and in some countries such as the UK and China, they show food intake falling whereas aggregate food availability is increasing. It is probable that there is an increasing proportion of waste as intake and income rise, but unlikely that the marginal propensity to waste food is higher than one—so it is hard to believe that actual consumption falls while availability (or purchases) increases. The other possible explanation is that household survey data could increasingly underestimate actual intake over time: the level of underreporting increases among the overweight, therefore as average weight increases so does the level of underreporting of consumption; and meals outside the home are frequently excluded from surveys, but even if not, there is evidence that food from meals eaten outside the home is more under-reported than food eaten at home. The share of food eaten outside the home is everywhere increasing. The gap between energy availability and energy intake from surveys is also much larger than expected, for example in the UK availability is 3,400 calories per person per day, whereas survey data record an intake of only 2,100 calories. The authors have found no explanation for these incompatibilities, particularly the divergent trends.

Table 1.3. Changes in calorie availability in different world areas, 1990–2005

Country	1990	2000	2005	Change 1990–2005 (%)
United Kingdom	3,206	3,370	3,449	+7.6
United States of America	3,576	3,815	3,690	+3.2
Africa	2,358	2,370	2,452	+4.0
Eastern Africa	1,951	2,008	2,007	+2.9
Middle Africa	2,106	1,832	1,840	−12.6
Northern Africa	2,935	3,006	3,142	+7.1
Southern Africa	2,666	2,598	2,770	+3.9
Western Africa	2,372	2,464	2,640	+11.3
America	3,050	3,228	3,255	+6.7
Northern America	3,530	3,794	3,685	+4.4
Central America	3,020	2,975	3,063	+1.4
Latin America, Caribbean	2,741	2,882	2,997	+9.3
Caribbean	2,426	2,519	2,724	+12.3
Asia	2,578	2,675	2,763	+7.2
Central Asia	3,051	2,441	2,541	−16.7
Eastern Asia	2,728	2,886	2,982	+9.3
Southern Asia	2,407	2,458	2,510	+4.3
Southeastern Asia	2,496	2,729	2,944	+17.9
Western Asia	2,661	2,618	2,660	−0.0
Europe	3,348	3,284	3,407	+1.7
Eastern Europe	3,314	3,060	3,377	+1.9
Northern Europe	3,224	3,344	3,398	+5.4
Southern Europe	3,201	3,335	3,276	+2.3
Western Europe	3,592	3,585	3,564	−0.8
Oceania	2,927	3,107	2,966	+1.3
Australia and New Zealand	3,095	3,336	3,149	+1.7
Melanesia	2,315	2,360	2,381	+2.8
Micronesia	2,561	2,841	2,996	+17.0
Polynesia	2,897	3,115	3,149	+8.7
World	2,723	2,784	2,859	+5.0
European Union 27	3,437	3,490	3,517	+2.3
Least developed countries	2,084	2,119	2,192	+5.2
World developed countries	3,339	3,368	3,418	+2.3
World developing countries	2,552	2,642	2,731	+7.0

Source: FAO Statistical databases (FAOSTAT), <http://www.fao.org/corp/statistics/en/>.

Turning to the energy expenditure side of the equation, good data are unavailable and past trends are usually explored through proxy variables, like nature of employment, television viewing, walking, cycling, and car ownership. In part, a reduction in energy expenditure can be attributed to economic development. People become less active as an economy evolves from agriculture, associated with physical labor, to heavy manufacturing industry, also associated with high levels of physical labor, to an economy dominated by light manufacturing industry and services, associated with low levels of physical activity.

Economic development is also associated with the process of urbanization as people move from the countryside to towns and cities. Urbanization is generally taken to mean lower energy expenditure in shopping and in leisure. People walk less, they have greater access to public transport, and drive cars. Interestingly, some counterevidence from the US shows that obesity is *lower* in urban areas, even after controlling for income and other likely differences between urban and rural inhabitants. Possible explanations include greater availability of gyms, a higher probability of walking to work than in rural areas of the US, and possibly greater health consciousness.[22] Finally, as people grow richer, they buy televisions and computers, so leisure becomes less physical.[23]

In developing countries these changes are arguably causing a substantial decrease in average energy expenditure, although we do not know exactly how much. In developed countries, however, much of the change in the structure of employment had already taken place by the time obesity rates started to grow sharply. Table 1.4 shows that although change continues, already by 1990 considerably less than 10% of the population of high-income countries was employed in agriculture and a further fifth to a third in industry, the remainder in services.

Regarding travel, data for Great Britain over the period 1975–2004 (Table 1.5) show a marked increase in the number of miles traveled per person, roughly 43%, but miles walked decreased by almost one quarter and miles cycled by about 30%, while car miles went up by more than 60%.

Data for physical activity during leisure are difficult to obtain and rarely comparable across countries, but there are indications that in many developed countries levels have risen over the past twenty years. Figure 1.3 shows trends in the proportion of people with 'inadequate physical activity' (based on slightly different definitions) in the US, UK, and Italy. This figure highlights how the situation has slightly improved in the Anglo-Saxon countries, while countries like Italy are experiencing a rising level of inadequate activity.

Bleich et al. (2007) have collected data from several sources to divide the cause of changes in obesity in some developed countries between energy intake and energy expenditure. They conclude that although physical activity has declined, the magnitude of the change explains little of the change in adult obesity except in Australia and Finland; they attribute almost all the change in obesity in other countries to increased calorie

----

[22] Mandal and Chern (2006).   [23] Popkin (2001).

Table 1.4. Structure of employment and urbanization in selected countries, 1990–2001

	Agriculture (%) 1990	2001	Industry (%) 1990	2001	Services (%) 1990	2001	Urban population 1990	2001
Argentina	0.4	0.8	31.6	21.9	67.6	76.9	87.0	89.4
Australia	6.5	4.9	25.0	20.9	69.5	74.1	85.4	87.4
Bangladesh	66.4	62.1	13.0	10.3	16.2	23.5	19.8	23.6
Brazil	22.8	20.6	22.7	20.0	54.5	59.4	74.8	81.8
Cameroon	60.6	60.6	9.1	9.1	23.1	23.1	40.7	50.9
Canada	4.3	2.9	24.4	22.7	71.3	74.4	76.6	79.5
Chile	19.3	13.6	25.2	23.9	55.5	62.5	83.3	86.2
China	53.4	45.2	19.0	17.3	9.9	12.7	27.4	36.7
Finland	8.9	5.6	30.4	27.2	60.5	66.7	61.4	61.1
Italy	8.9	5.3	32.3	32.1	58.8	62.5	66.7	67.3
Japan	7.2	4.9	34.1	30.5	58.2	63.9	63.1	65.3
Korea, Republic of	17.9	10.0	35.4	27.5	46.7	62.5	73.8	79.8
Mexico	22.6	17.6	27.8	26.0	39.6	56.0	72.5	75.0
Peru	1.2	8.8	27.3	17.9	71.5	73.3	68.9	71.8
Switzerland	4.2	4.2	32.2	26.2	63.6	69.6	68.4	73.5
Turkey	46.9	37.6	20.7	22.7	32.4	39.7	59.2	65.2
UK	1.1	1.4	32.4	24.9	66.2	73.4	88.7	89.5
US	2.9	2.4	26.2	22.4	70.9	75.2	75.3	79.4
High income: OECD	6.2	4.0	30.0	26.5	63.6	69.3	73.3	76.1
Latin America and Caribbean	16.3	17.3	25.9	21.4	55.8	61.2	71.0	75.7
Lower middle income	49.9	42.1	18.6	18.0	16.8	22.3	35.1	43.3

Source: World Development Indicators (2008), <http://go.worldbank.org/U0FSM7AQ40>.

Table 1.5. Average miles traveled per year by mode of travel, Great Britain, 1975/1976–2004

Mode of travel	1975 1976	1985 1986	1992 1994	1998 2000	2002	2003	2004	Change 1975–2004 (%)
Walk	255	244	199	192	189	192	196	−23.14
Bicycle	51	44	38	39	33	34	36	−29.41
Private hire bus	150	131	110	107	124	135	131	−12.67
Car, van driver	1,971	2,425	3,205	3,560	3,555	3,465	3,469	+76.0
Car, van passenger	1,401	1,600	2,030	2,011	2,065	2,048	1,999	+42.7
Motorcycle, moped	47	51	32	30	33	36	34	−27.66
Other private vehicles	16	33	43	26	20	27	22	+37.5
Bus in London	57	39	42	40	42	51	50	−12.28
Other local bus	372	258	217	205	214	213	206	−44.62
Non-local bus	54	109	96	99	58	86	75	+38.9
London Underground	36	44	50	57	62	54	51	+41.7
Surface rail	289	292	298	371	373	347	384	+32.9
Taxi, minicab	13	27	38	58	55	49	49	+276.9
Other public (air, ferries, light rail, etc.)	18	22	41	45	56	96	64	+255.6
All modes	4,740	5,317	6,439	6,840	6,879	6,833	6,762	+42.7

Source: Department for Transport, National Travel Surveys 2001 and 2004, <htpp://www.dft.gov.uk/pgr/statistics/datatablespublications/personal/mainresults/>.

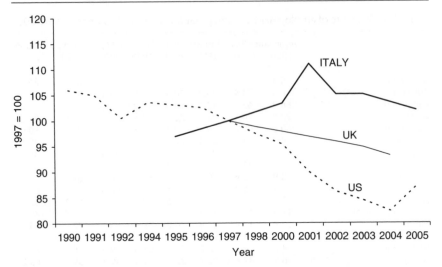

F<small>IG</small>. 1.3. Trends in the proportion of people with inadequate physical activity, standardized index (1997 = 100) for the US, UK, and Italy, 1990–2005

Definitions of inadequate physical activity differ by country and are as follows: US: no reported leisure time physical activities (i.e. any physical activities or exercises such as running, calisthenics, golf, gardening, or walking) in the previous month; UK: not meeting the target of a minimum of 30 minutes of at least moderate-intensity activity (such as brisk walking, cycling, or climbing the stairs) on five or more days of the week; Italy: no reported leisure time physical activities.

Sources: Our processing on data from the US Center for Disease Control and Prevention, UK Department of Health, and Italian National Institute of Statistics, various years.

intake. This is a controversial conclusion. Food intake data from household surveys in some countries including Britain have shown a declining trend,[24] suggesting that reduction in energy expenditure may be responsible for growing obesity. But household data are subject to underreporting, especially for snacking, eating out, and alcohol consumption, which have increased over the last decade. Also the obese are known to be more likely to underreport food intake. Reasons for divergent trends in per capita availability from aggregate data and intake from household data need further investigation, but the balance of evidence supports greater energy intake as causing weight gain over time.

Obesity is not the only cause of diet-related ill health; an unbalanced diet can also be harmful. For example, too much saturated fat has an impact on low- and high-density lipoprotein levels (LDL and HDL) in

---

[24] See e.g. Chesher (1997) on British data.

the blood,[25] which has been linked to blood pressure, heart disease, and stroke; fruit and vegetables have protective roles against some cancers; and salt is a factor in hypertension. Although our main focus is on issues concerning excess weight, we would be remiss not to mention these other aspects of diet, especially since they tend to become intertwined with weight control and general healthy eating messages emanating from governments. For example, the recommendation to eat more fruit and vegetables is partly because of their direct role in protecting against cancer and partly because they do not have many calories per gram compared to other foods (what is called low energy density). If you eat a lot of fruit and vegetables, you have less room in your stomach for high energy density foods with a lot of calories per gram, mainly fatty and sugary foods, e.g. soft drinks.

The Food and Agriculture Organization (FAO) and WHO held an expert consultation in 2002.[26] Based on this meeting, they generated several population-level nutrient intake recommendations, some of which have proven controversial, notably that calories from sugar should not exceed 10% of total calorie intake. The sugar lobby, particularly in the US, tried (and failed) to have the recommendation removed, claiming a lack of scientific evidence of a link between the calorie share from sugar and any health effects. Other key recommendations from the consultation include consumption of more than 400 grams of fruit and vegetables per day, and less than 30% of energy intake to come from fat and less than 10% from saturated fatty acids.[27]

Schmidhuber and Shetty (2005) have charted changes in dietary composition associated with the nutrition transition. They show that in 1962,

---

[25] HDL is known as good cholesterol, LDL as bad cholesterol. A poor fatty acid balance can lead to excess levels of LDL in the blood.

[26] WHO (2003).

[27] As a slight divergence we reiterate that these are population targets, but they tend to be treated by governments as individual targets. Take fruit and vegetables and assume for simplicity a symmetrical distribution of consumption through the population; then implicitly if the 400 grams target was exactly met, half of the population would consume less than 400 grams. One would presume, in setting a target, the FAO–WHO consultants would have in mind a healthy level of consumption, say 200 grams per day, and an estimate of the variance of consumption around the mean, and that the 400 gram recommendation was chosen so that only a small proportion of the population, say 1%, fell into the lower tail of the distribution with consumption less than two 200 grams per day. We have asked nutritionists about this and it is not how they think or interpret the recommendation, nor is it how government healthy eating messages treat the target. In both cases they recommend people consume (at least) 400 grams of fruit and vegetables per day. For example, the UK Food Standards Agency's healthy eating recommendations advise the consumption of at least five 80 gram portions of fruit and vegetables per day. Our point is not that either the FAO–WHO population recommendation or the individual recommendation is wrong, merely that they are inconsistent.

based on data for 158 countries, twenty-eight had more than the recommended 30% maximum of energy from fat and forty-seven more than the recommended 10% maximum of energy from saturated-fat consumption; by 2000, of 178 countries, sixty-one and sixty-two exceeded the two fat targets. The increases are largely associated with animal foods; in 1962 developing countries consumed on average 117 calories per person per day from livestock products and by 1998 this figure had more than doubled to 284. They project the figure to rise to 393 by 2030. Industrialized countries already consumed 670 calories per person per day from livestock products in 1962, 786 in 1998, and the figure is projected to rise to 847 by 2030.

There are positive signs that developed countries are taking the healthy eating message seriously. An examination of EU diets since the 1960s shows that the richer northern countries reduced their high levels of consumption of sugar and fats, particularly saturated fats, to levels nearer (albeit still slightly above) the FAO–WHO recommendations. In 1961 more than half of EU countries had fruit and vegetable availability below 400 grams per person per day, but by 2003 fruit and vegetable availability exceeded the recommendation in all fifteen (as it was then) EU countries, though given high levels of waste from these products, actual consumption still fell below the recommendation in some of them.[28]

Recently, two studies have looked into the changes in dietary pattern in relation to the WHO guidelines.[29] Figure 1.4 shows the evolution of a synthetic indicator of distance from the 'ideal' WHO diet for a selection of OECD countries. Exact compliance with guidelines would give an index value of 1. Diets show a clear tendency to improvement, which is stronger in higher-income areas. The graph suggests that UK and US diets, which were the worst in the 1960s, have progressively improved toward the WHO recommendations. In contrast, the 'Mediterranean' countries of Italy, France, Spain, and Greece drifted away from their near 'perfect' diet at the start of the period and by the end were little 'better' than the US or UK. We should highlight the fact that the WHO guidelines do not include a recommendation for calorie intake. Therefore, a 'perfect' diet by this definition (index = 1) can still involve too many calories consumed in relation to calorie expenditure. Clearly this is what has happened in the US and the UK: the composition of diets (also known as diet quality) has improved but the level of consumption has been too high, leading to increased obesity rates.

---

[28] Schmidhuber and Traill (2006).
[29] Schmidhuber and Traill (2006); Mazzocchi et al. (2007).

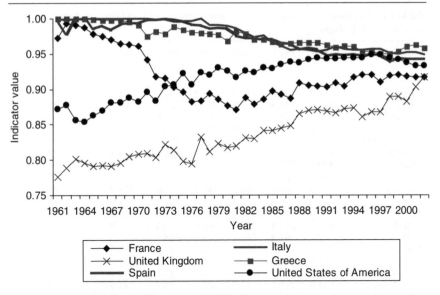

FIG. **1.4.** Indicator of compliance with WHO dietary recommendations (1 = perfect compliance) in selected OECD countries, 1961–2002

Source: Mazzocchi et al. (2008).

Health Trends

The evidence suggests that weight gains in the developed world can be blamed on increased calorie intake, although diet quality has shown signs of improvement in other respects. Governments are concerned that the greater weight will adversely impact health. The dangers are well known: increased risk of heart disease, type II diabetes, stroke (through hypertension), and certain cancers. One would anticipate finding increasing death rates from these illnesses since the 1980s, when rates of obesity started to climb sharply. Comparable international health data are available only for OECD countries and they refer only to mortality rates from various diseases, not to prevalence of the disease itself. By far the highest mortality rate associated with diet-related non-communicable diseases (NCDs) is from heart disease. Table 1.6 shows that in 2000 the average mortality rate among reporting OECD countries was about 120 per 100,000 population compared to less than 10 per 100,000 population for diabetes. The death rate from heart disease has almost halved in OECD countries from its peak in the late 1960s. The variation among countries has also decreased dramatically. In the late 1960s the mortality rate was above 300 per 100,000 in Australia, Canada, Finland, and the United States but below

Table 1.6. Mortality rates from ischemic heart disease per 100,000 population in OECD countries, 1960–2004

	1960	1970	1980	1990	2000	2004	Change 1960–2004 (%)
Australia	338.0	345.8	242.5	179.3	108.0	91.3[a]	−73
Austria	232.8	198.3	147.1	147.3	125.3	104.5[b]	−55
Belgium	130.5	158.4	126.0	83.9	79.0[c]		
Canada	351.8	309.4	231.8	154.2	108.5	97.2[d]	−72
Czech Republic				297.0	179.1	155.6	
Denmark	269.4	276.9	261.2	201.6	106.0	106.4[e]	−61
Finland	330.8	293.8	265.2	229.5	167.7	137.2	−59
France	74.4	69.5	73.5	59.5	46.8	42.5[a]	−43
Germany	204.3	156.2	162.2	147.4	121.0	104.2	−49
Greece	102.3	66.4	76.3	91.8	82.8	82.9	−19
Hungary	259.5	239.4	217.0	226.6	214.8	219.7[a]	−15
Iceland	201.3	262.1	224.5	166.4	116.8	106.0	−47
Ireland	319.4	267.3	264.9	228.5	158.7	107.6[b]	−66
Italy	232.7	140.1	123.2	90.4	70.2	68.5[d]	−71
Japan	91.0	60.0	52.0	36.5	33.4	29.5	−68
Korea, Republic of				17.3	32.0	34.9	
Luxembourg	163.0	215.1	137.7	103.4	78.7	72.5	−56
Mexico		54.0		92.6	106.2[f]		
Netherlands	215.9	199.5	167.2	125.9	82.8	61.5	−72
New Zealand	308.2	303.9	277.2	200.5	129.7	133.4[e]	−57
Norway	211.1	230.0	200.6	180.4	110.9	84.6	−60
Poland	81.0	77.0	101.5	112.3	133.4	110.9	+37
Portugal	136.9	162.1	89.6	79.6	59.9	59.4[a]	−57
Slovak Republic					278.5	266.8[d]	
Spain	93.0		75.1	70.5	62.3	54.5	−41
Sweden	276.9	280.1	276.8	179.2	118.0	112[d]	−60
Switzerland	265.1	107.2	115.6	105.6	86.8	67.5	−75
United Kingdom	302.9	254.0	247.7	207.2	129.7[e]	108.7	−64
United States	374.0	362.0	237.1	166.7	139.6	127.6[d]	−66

[a] Data for 2003.   [b] Data for 2005.   [c] Data for 1997.   [d] Data for 2002.   [e] Data for 2001.
[f] Data for 1995.

Source: OECD Health Data (2007), <http://oberon.sourceoecd.org>.

100 in France, Japan, Spain, and Mexico. By 1980 it had already fallen sharply, though twelve countries still had mortality rates above 200 per 100,000 (eight between 100 and 200 per 100,000, five below 100 per 100,000). By 2000 only the new member countries Hungary and the Slovak Republic reported mortality rates above 200 per 100,000 population but among the old member countries only Finland had mortality rates above 130 per 100,000 and eleven were below 100 per 100,000. Similar trends are observable for other NCDs.

Could this mean that obesity reduces deaths from heart disease? No, the negative effect of obesity on mortality has been offset by the positive effects of reduced prevalence of smoking, improvements in medical technology, more and better medical screening, more resources devoted to treatment. Today it has never been safer to be overweight, which suggests that warnings to lose weight for health may be ineffective if people are aware of the true risks.

Without entering into the biological debate, we note that the relationship between BMI and life expectancy is not clear-cut. Tucker et al. (2006) show that in the US life expectancy among 20-year-olds falls, as expected, as BMI increases; for example, it is about six years longer at age 20 for a BMI of 24 than for a BMI of 44. In older people, the relationship is less clear-cut; at age 60, life expectancy for white females is maximized at a BMI of 27–9 and among black males and females life expectancy *increases* right up to a BMI of 44. Only for white males is life expectancy maximized at a BMI of 24–6 and even then it falls by only three years with a BMI of 44. As obesity is strongly associated with age and social status, so, it seems, are the health consequences of obesity. This again suggests that interventions targeted at overweight and obese categories may be inadequate as policy guides as age, race, and other socio-demographic factors should be considered in making targeted interventions to reduce obesity. This holds if the subgroups of the population are motivated differently; it is important to discover their separate motivations and intervene appropriately.

Good health goes beyond life expectancy; the quality of life also matters. Evidence cited in the UK's Foresight Report[30] states that the relative risk of diabetes for men with BMI 31–3 is forty times greater than for BMI <25. Diabetes is a disease with serious side-effects[31] and the prevalence of type II has increased around the world. The world prevalence of diabetes (all ages) was 2.8% in 2000, and is projected to rise to 4.4% in 2030. In developed countries, type II diabetes prevalence is expected to reach 6.8% in 2030, with peaks above 10% in Greece, Spain, and Italy.[32] Relative risks for other diseases are not so dramatic; obesity increases the risk of heart disease and stroke by about 20% in men and women and it also raises the risk of a number of cancers and arthritis.[33] Figure 1.5 shows increasing trends in morbidity rates for circulatory diseases[34] in Great Britain.

---

[30] Foresight 'creates challenging visions of the future to ensure effective strategies now'; see McPherson et al. (2007).

[31] For an account of the medical problems associated with diabetes in the US, see e.g. Kleinfield, 'Living at an Epicenter of Diabetes, Defiance and Despair', *New York Times*, 9 Jan. 2006.

[32] See Wild et al. (2004) and projections in the appendix, <http://care.diabetesjournals.org/content/vol27/issue5/images/data/1047/DC1/Wild_Appendix.xls>.

[33] See McPherson et al. (2007).

[34] According to the official WHO classification, 'diseases of the circulatory system' include acute rheumatic fever, chronic rheumatic heart diseases, hypertensive diseases, ischemic heart

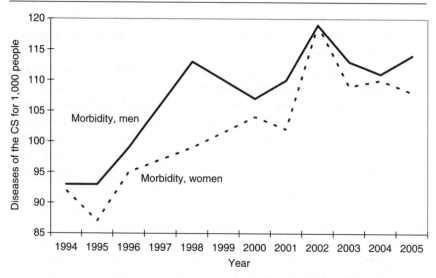

FIG. 1.5. Rates per 1,000 population reporting long-standing diseases of the circulatory system (CS) by sex, Great Britain, 1994–2005

Source: Department of Health (2007), 'Trends in Prevalence of All CHD', <http://www.heartstats.org/datapage.asp?id=1617>.

Our main message in this brief review of data is that the relationships between eating, exercise, weight, and disease may be well known scientifically, but it is less clear when one considers real-world data in which human behavior interacts with food, obesity, and health. There are significant unexplained differences across countries and, within countries, subgroups of the population vary in BMI and its health consequences. Some reasons are biological, but some are behavioral. Economics provides additional insight into these behavioral challenges, and it is these we focus on throughout the book.

Why Are People Eating More? The Need to Understand Behavior as well as Biology

Economists believe in the existence of consumer sovereignty. This means that, in studying diets, economists take on a useful and necessary fiction: we assume that people in active exchange institutions like a market make

diseases, pulmonary heart disease and diseases of pulmonary circulation, other forms of heart disease, cerebrovascular diseases, diseases of arteries, arterioles, and capillaries, diseases of veins, lymphatic vessels, and lymph nodes (not elsewhere classified), and other and unspecified disorders of the circulatory system.

decisions that maximize their utility (or satisfaction or happiness). People derive utility from all sorts of goods and services bought and sold on the marketplace: drink, food, cars, holidays, iPods—the list is almost limitless. Their resources to buy them, however, are finite, so people must make choices on how to spend their incomes. Since everyone's preferences are their own and people have different incomes, they all choose different combinations of goods and services to maximize utility. Over time, as incomes change or the prices of goods change, they make different choices even if their preferences are unchanged. This viewpoint provides a useful mindset to frame how people make choices in a market setting. Economists know the world is more complex—but their framework provides a rational benchmark against which to compare actual behavior within a market and to assess directions of change in response to external stimuli and the ways in which decision variables interact with one another as choices are made.

The basic benchmark model can be extended in many ways; for example, the notion that people have a given income and they decide how best to spend it is misleading when viewed over a lifetime because they can invest in education or work hard to become more productive and better paid in the future. They also have some flexibility in how many hours to work, allowing them to convert leisure time into income. These decisions also depend on preferences—how much people are prepared to forsake present consumption in favor of future consumption (what economists call the time preference or discount rate) and how they value income relative to leisure. People also gain utility from non-market intangibles like their health and appearance, which are affected by overeating. This can be counteracted by exercise or by buying better health insurance. If advances in medical technology and higher levels of health expenditure by governments make being overweight less dangerous (we have seen that the effect of obesity on mortality has diminished), people may decide not to give up as much current consumption of unhealthy but tasty food and so they might eat more and become fatter. We see how understanding behavior becomes complicated when we admit that health, incomes, the amount of leisure, the amount of exercise, and the amount and types of food people eat and their weight are all interrelated—they are endogenous.

In their basic form, economic decision models assume people know the relationships between the key variables and know their own minds. They make consumption and leisure choices in a market setting to maximize utility in every time period subject to constraints on the amount of time in a day and their genetic endowments of health, wisdom, and beauty. But even if the typical person does not make these complex calculations in reality, economists expect that decisions will be taken to increase utility, even if not maximize it. Theoretical models thus help to frame choice, so economists can gain more understanding about which variables are related to one another and in which direction people respond to some external shock to the system. Given the proper data, our empirical models can measure the strength of the response, if not at the individual level, then for a country or a socio-economic group within a country. For instance, a basic economic prediction is that, as prices go up, people demand less of the good, and our empirical models can estimate the strength of the response.

But additional complications arise. Most decisions we take are clouded in uncertainty: although being obese increases the risk of a range of diseases, it might not apply to me as an individual given my genetics and exercise habits. How I, as an individual, react to the risk depends on how I judge or misjudge the likelihood I'll be one of the lucky ones who 'gets away with it' and upon my attitude to risk—how risk averse am I? More importantly, are there certain groups in society who are more risk averse or more skilled at risk reduction than others and why, and are there some cultures more risk averse or skilled than others? Can this explain differences in behavior toward diet and health? Are certain risks systematically under- or overrated through the population and is behavior affected (e.g. most people think they are better than average car drivers and less likely to have an accident)? Is the risk of being obese overestimated because the information people receive from newspapers, television, nutritionists, and doctors is alarmist, whereas data suggest mortality rates from diet-related ill health have been falling? People make decisions based on their perceptions of risks rather than the objective facts.

This is our economist's mindset as we write this book—we view obesity as a matter of choice. Why have people chosen to be more overweight now than they were twenty years ago? Our answer to this question differs from the biology-driven answer. They choose to frame their answer by talking about the creation of an exogenous *obesogenic environment* in which people cannot help but get fat. To this way of thinking the food industry is to blame for making unhealthy foods and persuading us to eat them, super-sized; and government is to blame for subsidizing farmers to produce unhealthy industrialized foods. In contrast, our economic perspective makes these choices endogenous. Nowadays, in all but the poorest countries, people do have real choice. Nothing compels us to go out and buy a Big Mac with jumbo fries and a pint of coke.

A supermarket is likely to be nearby selling fresh fruit and vegetables and all the other ingredients for a delicious home-cooked meal. The home-cooked meal might cost more and take more time, and people might *choose* to eat the unhealthy option and use their money and time on other things.

We believe it is important to establish with a certain degree of formality the parameters involved in a person's individual decision making, and we do this in the next chapter. The formal structure helps to explain why some people, or groups of people, *choose* to be more overweight than others, and more overweight than in the past. The structure also helps to inform policy interventions which should be targeted at the specific behavioral causes of obesity in the target group.

What Does This Have to Do with Governments?

Private citizens do not make perfect choices, but they do the best they can for themselves—better than by bureaucratic fiat from London, Rome, or Washington. This is a popular view among the public, and many economists share this view. But there are two basic reasons economists support government intervention in what would otherwise be a personal choice: the decision about how much you weigh.

First, we must consider whether people are sufficiently educated and informed. Information provided by manufacturers can be one-sided. Economists concede government has a role to play in ensuring that information is fair and reasonably complete and people know enough to act on it if they want to. Children may be susceptible to misleading messages or to an attractive sales pitch. Neither can they be expected to take the long view and forsake current pleasure for the sake of a future well-being beyond their perception, so they may be a special case. Protecting children leads to a call for 'protection' from advertising of junk foods and soft drinks or their provision in vending machines in schools. We argue, though, that a policy response should be based on good evidence of harm, not just a supposition, and it should be proportionate: the benefits of intervention should outweigh the costs. This is true of all interventions and is a major element throughout the book.

Economists' other rationale for governments to overrule freedom of individual choice is when one person's choices harm others. This is called 'market failure' or an 'externality'. Although passive obesity is a less likely cause of harm to others than passive smoking, the main economic problem lies in who receives the health bill when a person becomes ill from overeating. If it is the individual, health care costs would be figured into his or her utility-maximizing decision: being fat would be a risk to health and a costly one. In reality, in all developed countries, health is publicly funded to some degree. The cost burden is then redistributed across all taxpayers. There are conceptual issues surrounding the calculation and interpretation of these costs and we return to them in more detail in Chapter 3.

Another challenge for economists is to quantify the 'indirect' costs of reduced productivity due to obesity. Are 'heavier' people less productive at work? Do they miss more working days because of obesity-related health problems? While medical progress has reduced the risk of obesity-related mortality in developed countries, evidence is that obesity reduces labor productivity and leads to significant increases in lost working days. Again, employment law means this cost is borne by society or the employer. Some authors further suggest additional costs could be imputed to decreased opportunities in education, housing, and employment because of societal blame of the obese.[35]

Health Inequalities

Obesity and its health problems are most common among those who are already deprived, typically those in lower socio-economic groups and, in America, blacks and Latinos. Many hypotheses for this could be put forward, some of them politically incorrect, some perhaps overly politically correct: that people in these groups lack self-control; they are undereducated and do not understand nutritional labels; healthy food is too expensive for poor people so they have to rely on cheap calories from processed and fast foods; they have different social norms—the pressures to be thin are greatest for the ambitious middle classes;[36] blacks, native American Indians, and perhaps Latinos have inherited a 'thrifty gene' which makes them efficient at storing food as fat during a food shortage (of evolutionary benefit) but predisposes them to overweight in times of plenty;[37] supermarkets have closed down most of the cheap, small local shops so those who do not own a car rely on the few local shops remaining

---

[35] Hutton (1994).
[36] See Oliver (2006: 74–6).
[37] Schmidhuber and Shetty (2005).

and these do not sell healthy food like fruit and vegetables; only the better off can afford gym membership.

The list could go on, and what is interesting is that each hypothesis can be framed in an economic context to define a testable empirical hypothesis—if the data are available or can be collected. Also, each suggests a different policy response. Policy is not evidence-based if it does not proceed in this way, but many of the advocates of one hypothesis or another seem prepared to propose government policy intervention without any evidence or with anecdotal evidence: data can be the enemy of many a good theory.

Action Always Has Costs to Go with the Benefits

If there are market failures, one may argue for government action.[38] But this is true in part: any intervention has costs and benefits. From an economist's perspective, the benefits must outweigh the costs. The direct costs of nutritional labeling, including analysis, quality control, and printing of labels, are borne by food manufacturers and retailers, but in the long run they can be passed on to consumers in the form of higher food prices. There may be differential impacts on small and large firms because many of the costs are fixed (independent of the amount produced), meaning that proportionately the rise in costs per unit are higher for small firms, which may make them uncompetitive; for example, many small abattoirs in Europe have been driven out of business by stringent EU meat safety regulations.[39] Since governments believe the protection of small firms is also a key policy objective, this may be seen as a cost of regulation.

In Chapter 4 we discuss an array of policy interventions available to affect food choice and obesity, ranging from information interventions such as nutritional labeling, advertising restrictions, social marketing, fat taxes and thin subsidies, legal liability, and many more. In each case we discuss what data are needed to evaluate the policy and present existing empirical evidence.

Measuring and comparing costs and benefits is a challenge. How can one address questions such as how many small firms driven out of business equate to one life extended by a year? Economists argue it is at least

---

[38] More open to debate, but still widely accepted, is that it is also government's duty to reduce health inequalities. For example, this is explicitly stated as a policy objective of the UK Department of Health.

[39] Dunn (2003).

necessary to quantify all the costs and benefits and allow the political process to weigh the two and decide whether the balance favors legislation. This is rarely done in practice. Obtaining evidence itself incurs costs, as collecting and analyzing complex data is not cheap—and in some cases the benefits of obtaining evidence may themselves be outweighed by the costs. Data collection takes a serious commitment, especially given the long-term nature of diet, obesity, and health relationships. Government action is currently based on incomplete evidence.[40]

Conclusions

In this chapter we have examined the data on obesity, healthy eating, and health. In all OECD countries with the exception of Japan and Korea there has been an inexorable upward trend in adult and child obesity levels, a trend beginning around the 1980s. The trend is being replicated, at lower income levels, in the middle- and even lower-income countries. There have been, however, wide divergences in obesity levels across countries at similar stages of development which have not been satisfactorily explained by economic, cultural, or institutional variables.

A closer look at the distribution of obesity within a country reveals a rightward shift in which everyone over time has become heavier but there has also been a flattening of the distribution, as those in the right-hand tail of the distribution have put on weight faster than the population at large. There may be some biological susceptibility, but the obesity problem is most prevalent among disadvantaged groups, those of lower socioeconomic group, lower education, and, in America anyway, ethnic minorities; this suggests a behavioral explanation.

The biological cause of weight gain over time is higher energy intake than expenditure. Some people still debate whether increased intake or reduced expenditure or both are responsible; the balance of evidence, however, suggests increased intake is the primary culprit.

Many adverse health consequences are attributed to obesity: heart disease, stroke, diabetes, and several cancers. We have seen that, despite the dramatic increase in obesity, the death rate from these diseases has fallen in OECD countries, suggesting the mortality risk from being obese has fallen over the years; in many ways it is safer to be obese now than in the

[40] Wanless (2004).

past. We have also seen that, as with obesity, many non-communicable diseases associated with obesity are concentrated in disadvantaged groups.

Economics is a social science with a behavioral framework which can address questions of why people have become heavier over time, what are the consequences for resource allocation, and are policy interventions justifiable. Economics recognizes that what people eat and how much they exercise are bound up in broader questions of how they spend their time and money, and failure to recognize the complex interactions between biological and economic factors can lead to interventions which reduce rather than enhance people's welfare. We address these issues in the remainder of the book.

References

Anderson, P. M., K. F. Butcher, and P. B. Levine (2003), 'Economic Perspectives on Childhood Obesity', *Economic Perspectives*, 27/3: 30–49.

Bleich, S., D. M. Cutler, C. J. Murray, and A. Adams (2007), *Why Is the Developed World Obese?*, NBER Working Paper 12954.

Chesher, A. (1997), 'Diet Revealed? Semiparametric Estimation of Nutrient Intake Age Relationships', *Journal of the Royal Statistical Society Series A-Statistics in Society*, 160: 389–420.

Christakis, N. A., and J. H. Fowler (2007), 'The Spread of Obesity in a Large Social Network over 32 Years', *New England Journal of Medicine*, 357/4: 370–9.

Cole, T. J., M. C. Bellizzi, K. M. Flegal, and W. H. Dietz (2000), 'Establishing a Standard Definition for Child Overweight and Obesity Worldwide: International Survey', *British Medical Journal*, 320/7244: 1240–3.

Cutler, D. M., E. L. Glaeser, and J. M. Shapiro (2003), 'Why Have Americans Become More Obese?', *Journal of Economic Perspectives*, 17/3: 93–118.

Dhurandhar, N. V. (2001), 'Infectobesity: Obesity of Infectious Origin', *Journal of Nutrition*, 131/10: 2794S–2797S.

Dunn, E. C. (2003), 'Trojan Pig: Paradoxes of Food Safety Regulation', *Environment and Planning A*, 35/8: 1493–1511.

Finkelstein, E. A., I. C. Fiebelkorn, and G. J. Wang (2004), 'State-Level Estimates of Annual Medical Expenditures Attributable to Obesity', *Obesity Research*, 12/1: 18–24.

—— C. J. Ruhm, and K. M. Kosa (2005), 'Economic Causes and Consequences of Obesity', *Annual Review of Public Health*, 26: 239–57.

Fry, J., and W. Finley (2005), 'The Prevalence and Costs of Obesity in the EU', *Proceedings of the Nutrition Society*, 64/3: 359–62.

Harris, J. A., and F. G. Benedict (1918), 'A Biometric Study of Human Basal Metabolism', *Proceedings of the National Academy of Sciences*, 4/12: 370–3.

Hofstede, G. H. (2001), *Culture's Consequences: Comparing Values, Behaviors, Institutions, and Organizations Across Nations* (Thousand Oaks, Calif.: Sage Publications).

Hutton, J. (1994), 'The Economics of Treating Obesity', *Pharmacoeconomics*, 5: 66–72.

Kragelund, C., and T. Omland (2005), 'A Farewell to Body-Mass Index?', *The Lancet*, 366/9497: 1589–91.

Lang, T., and M. Heasman (2004), *Food Wars: The Global Battle for Mouths, Minds and Markets* (London: Earthscan).

Lobstein, T., and M. L. Frelut (2003), 'Prevalence of Overweight among Children in Europe', *Obesity Reviews*, 4: 195–200.

McPherson, K., T. Marsh, and M. Brown (2007), *Tackling Obesities: Future Choices: Modeling Future Trends in Obesity and the Impact on Health* (London: Government Office for Science).

Mandal, B., and W. Chern (2006), 'Changes in Factors Contributing to Rising Body Mass Index: 1997 versus 2002', *Consumer Interests Annual*, 52/6: 170–85.

Mazzocchi, M., C. Brasili, and E. Sandri (2008), 'Trends in Dietary Patterns and Compliance with World Health Organization Recommendations: A Cross-Country Analysis', *Public Health Nutrition*, 11/5: 535–40.

Mendez, M. A., and B. M. Popkin (2004), 'Globalization, Urbanization and Nutritional Change in the Developing World', *Electronic Journal of Agricultural and Development Economics*, 1/2: 220–41.

Oliver, J. E. (2006), *Fat Politics: The Real Story behind America's Obesity Epidemic* (New York: Oxford University Press).

Popkin, B. M. (2001), 'The Nutrition Transition and Obesity in the Developing World', *Journal of Nutrition*, 131/3: 871S–873S.

—— and S. W. Ng (2006), 'The Nutrition Transition in High- and Low-Income Countries: What Are the Policy Lessons?', International Association of Agricultural Economists Conference, Invited Paper, Gold Coast, Australia, 12–18 Aug.

Pulvers, K. M., R. E. Lee, H. Kaur, M. S. Mayo, M. L. Fitzgibbon, S. K. Jeffries, J. Butler, Q. Hou, and J. S. Ahluwalia (2004), 'Development of a Culturally Relevant Body Image Instrument among Urban African Americans', *Obesity Research*, 12/10: 1641–51.

Schmidhuber, J., and P. Shetty (2005), 'The Nutrition Transition to 2030: Why Developing Countries Are Likely to Bear the Major Burden', *Food Economics*, 2/3–4: 150–66.

—— and W. B. Traill (2006), 'The Changing Structure of Diets in the European Union in Relation to Healthy Eating Guidelines', *Public Health Nutrition*, 9/5: 584–95.

Thompson, D., J. B. Brown, G. A. Nichols, P. J. Elmer, and G. Oster (2001), 'Body Mass Index and Future Healthcare Costs: A Retrospective Cohort Study', *Obesity Research*, 9/3: 210–18.

Tucker, D. M. D., A. J. Palmer, W. J. Valentine, S. Roze, and J. A. Ray (2006), 'Counting the Costs of Overweight and Obesity: Modeling Clinical and Cost Outcomes', *Current Medical Research and Opinion*, 22/3: 575–86.

Wanless, D. (2004), *Securing Good Health for the Whole Population: Final Report* (Norwich: HMSO).

WHO (2003), *Diet, Nutrition and the Prevention of Chronic Diseases*, WHO Technical Report Series 916 (Geneva: World Health Organization).

—— (2004), *Food and Health in Europe: A New Basis for Action*, WHO Regional Publications European Series 96 (Copenhagen: World Health Organization Europe).

Wild, S., G. Roglic, A. Green, R. Sicree, and H. King (2004), 'Global Prevalence of Diabetes: Estimates for the Year 2000 and Projections for 2030', *Diabetes Care*, 27/5: 1047–53.

Wolf, A. M., and G. A. Colditz (1998), 'Current Estimates of the Economic Cost of Obesity in the United States', *Obesity Research*, 6/2: 97–106.

2

Why Obesity? An Economic Perspective

Chapter 1 defined the conventional thinking about today's obesity challenge. We now consider the economic perspective on obesity. We explore how the economic mindset can help us to understand better why we have witnessed more overweight people and obesity since the mid-1980s; why cross-country differences in obesity rates exist; and why the lower social and income classes are more obese on average. Our economic-based explanations can seem counterintuitive, conflicting with the conventional rationale. When possible, we provide empirical evidence to support the economic viewpoint.

We begin by addressing *the* fundamental economic question: is obesity a failure of the market economy? We examine the economic conditions when the answer is 'no' and when it is 'yes'. We then add more scientific rigor to our economic story. We define a model of consumer choice for food in a market economy. This allows us to go beyond speculation; rather, we generate testable hypotheses about what causes obesity in the developed world. Next we consider whether poor information in a market economy is a contributor to obesity. Finally, we discuss the implications for developing countries and children.

Is Obesity a Failure of the Market Economy?

Markets exist for all types of foods, healthy and unhealthy (e.g. carrots to chips). Markets also exist to improve one's health: markets for gyms, medicine, bicycles, health services, weight-loss clinics, and health insurance. Economists believe that markets are a good idea, one of the best ever discovered by humans. Markets are so useful because they coordinate cost-effectively all our decentralized tastes, technology, and resources. Consumers, producers, middlemen, and sellers can all gain by trading goods and services defined by property rights protected by a government. The power of the marketplace rests in its ability to allow people to trade such that goods and services move from low-value uses to higher-value uses.

The *market price* is the key. Economists see prices as more than 'what you pay for something'. Rather, prices are information. They reveal information on the relative scarcity of the good or service based on the classic idea of 'supply and demand'. If people demand more of a good, the price increases. Producers respond to these high prices by expanding production. If supply increases, prices fall to clear the market. *Market interaction* is the key to understand how prices change and how people respond in turn. Consumers substitute more expensive goods with cheaper goods; in response, suppliers might change what goods they offer. Economics makes the point that when markets work, they work well owing to this market interaction: this interaction generates market prices, which create the incentives for individuals to make private decisions that ultimately maximize the net benefits to society.

This is Adam Smith's classic 'invisible hand' of the market. If the key conditions to support a well-functioning market exist, economists believe that markets should be left alone and the final market equilibrium would reflect the best possible outcome for society. People achieve the best outcome through self-interest regulated by competition. It is important to acknowledge that in a perfectly operating market people can and do make private decisions that result in them becoming overweight or obese. Under such circumstances, economists see no case for government intervention.

But markets can fail. When a market fails, the equilibrium prices and quantities do not capture the total social costs and benefits. Goods impose costs on others without any compensation; other goods generate benefits to everyone regardless of whether they paid. When markets fail, economists argue that governmental intervention can rebalance private desires and social goals. Economists need first to check that a market failure exists, understand why, and evaluate which policy intervention might work to correct the failure cost-effectively.

Now let us put this abstract discussion of the market and market failure in the context of the obesity challenge. If markets are complete and working properly, people should not worry about other people being obese. Informed adults should have the freedom and flexibility to trade their future health in favor of a more enjoyable lifestyle today, which might include a fatty diet and little physical activity. People can make their own self-interested choices in which they balance their own private benefits with their own private costs. No government intervention is needed because people have made their own decisions about diet and health based on personal preferences, budget constraints, and relative prices that arise in market-based exchange. These prices capture the social values associated with private decisions.

But if markets fail, current prices do not reflect social values associated with obesity and private health. The critical question becomes understanding how the market has failed, and what governments can do to realign private and social costs—without making things worse and without generating unintended consequences of otherwise well-aimed policies. We now review the three main reasons why markets could fail for the case of obesity, and why this could help to explain the increasing obesity rates.

First, markets fail due to *externalities*. An externality is the classic case of market failure. An externality exists when any given transaction generates extra costs to people and society who are not part of the transaction. If obesity generates health care costs which are paid by all taxpayers, this is a market failure. Here a person's private decision whether to eat more (and risk becoming obese) based on market prices is distorted because he does not pay the full costs of this choice. Rather, he underestimates the costs of his obesity because a fraction of the cost is paid by others through higher health service fees. This results in a market outcome in which there are more obese people than society would like if all costs were accounted for in private decisions. Externalities also arise when a market action generates societal benefits and those gaining from the benefits are not paying for them.

Information problems are a second type of market failure relevant to obesity. In a well-working market, full and accurate information is available to everyone. People are assumed to use this information when making decisions. From an economics standpoint, when people make voluntary and informed choices and all costs and benefits of these choices are accounted for within the market, there is no reason for government intervention. But if, say, sellers have more information than buyers about the relative safety of their food product, an *information asymmetry* exists. Now market prices do not accurately reflect the costs and benefits of the good being sold. For example, the courts upheld successful lawsuits against tobacco companies given that the industry withheld available scientific information on health hazards from smoking.[1] Sellers knew

---

[1] See Iida and Proctor (2004).

more than buyers, and they intentionally withheld the information that could have aided decision making (as in the tobacco example).

Third, a *lack of competition* leads to market failure. How the market is structured matters for proper pricing of goods and services, i.e. when one or a few firms control the market, as with monopolies and oligopolies, prices can be inflated. Market power can reduce consumer choices and product substitutability. A mature market like food seems unlikely to be affected by this sort of problem. But it is necessary to look closer at how consumers and firms make their choices. For example, marketing actions targeted at enhancing brand image aim at making branded products less substitutable.

Public health decisions can be improved if we understand when markets fail and we understand why private decisions differ from social goals. To do this properly, we must first understand what makes up a well-operating market. This approach defines an economic benchmark against which we can judge whether the obesity challenge justifies the case for public intervention.

Consumer Decision Making

We begin by defining a *representative consumer*: a consumer who weighs the costs and benefits of his decision making. Our representative consumer does not reflect any one person in particular; rather, this consumer captures the ideal of how a *fully informed* person would react to changes in market conditions and government intervention. We use our representative consumer as a straw man; he is a benchmark against which we can judge whether obesity is due to market failure or not.

Economists believe in the principle of consumer sovereignty: each person is free to make his own decisions about what to buy. He is better able to weigh up his preferred alternatives and choose combinations of products (e.g. bundles of goods) that satisfy his own unique preferences than any outsider. If a person has the time and money and desire to buy something, he will have the opportunity to exercise that desire. While this rules out people in hospitals, prisons, and maybe schools, it captures the environment of our representative consumer.

We assume that consumer sovereignty holds for our consumer. The representative consumer has preferences that follow a set of rules, also called *axioms*, which define what choices make sense—rational choices—

and which ones do not. For example, one axiom is that when a person can choose between two *bundles* of goods which are identical in all respects except that one bundle has more of one good than the other, he prefers the bundle with more to the bundle with less. For example, three bars of chocolate, two bottles of wine, and one Porsche is preferred to two bars of chocolate, two bottles of wine, and one Porsche.[2]

The consumer's preferences over the various goods and services can be represented by the classical concept of a *utility function*. A utility function relates the consumer's satisfaction to how much he chooses to consume of a bundle of goods and services. The consumer chooses this bundle of goods to *maximize* his satisfaction (i.e. his utility). The outcome is constrained by income and the relative prices of the available goods and services. Our consumer maximizes his utility given a budget constraint, which limits him to spending no more than he earns or borrows.

We used several assumptions to construct our representative consumer as a benchmark against which we can judge reality and empirical observation. First, our consumer knows his own preferences for a wide array of goods. In reality, we do not know how we feel about all goods and services since there are many. The goods and services available to the average consumer in a developed country run into the hundreds of thousands. Large Western supermarkets sell tens of thousands of food and drink items. Second, our consumer knows both the quality of all goods and their prices with certainty. Third, he 'acts as if' he can make the necessary calculations to decide if buying, say, a newspaper on the way to work will help to increase his satisfaction. Economists work with this necessary fiction because it provides the baseline against which we can judge market successes and failures. Our representative consumer approximates the way people behave within markets and helps to define the range of actual behavior.

While a reader may have raised an eyebrow thinking about potential problems of these assumptions, we ask you to remember that economic research has extended this benchmark consumer by including health status, risk and uncertainty, borrowing and saving, imperfect knowledge, habit formation, and so forth. The challenge is not to dismiss the ideal consumer as unrealistic, but to identify how a real consumer who makes choices in the marketplace compares to this benchmark. In doing so, you

---

[2] Other axioms are consistency and diminishing marginal utility: see any introductory microeconomics text such as Estrin and Laidler (1995).

can understand better the economic perspective: how do economic circumstances contribute to obesity; is obesity due to a real or imagined market failure; and does market failure validate government intervention into the food and health industries?

For example, consider one relevant extension to the obesity problem: treating time as a constraint on choices. Economists have argued that *time* not income is the only true constraint on human choice, because time can be converted to income by working. Adding a time constraint to our model takes it another step closer to the real choices people make about diet and health.[3] The time constraint extension implies that our representative consumer has more choices to make: how many hours to work, whether to buy fresh ingredients to prepare and cook at home, or prepared food from the supermarket, or to eat out, how much to eat, and how much to exercise. This extension is called the *household production function* (HHP) approach because it allows for households to allocate their time both to production activities (e.g. the production of meals) and to consumption activities, which we now discuss in more detail.[4]

The Household Production Function Approach

The household production model captures the wide range of substitutions and trade-offs consumers face in their everyday choices. The model assumes that consumer utility depends on choices over all goods and nonconsumption activities like leisure, and health status. In Box 2.1 we explain the HHP approach in greater detail as applied to obesity-related choices.

Box 2.1. The household production approach, obesity, and health

Suppose our consumer derives utility from eating, drinking, smoking (S), consumption of goods which do not affect health (Z), leisure (L), and the state of health (H). Both nature and nurture matter for state of health. Health is affected by nature: genetics and chance affect one's predisposition to obesity and ill health. Health is also affected by nurture: health depends on how we choose to live, e.g. smoking, drinking, and weight. The point is obvious: people *choose* whether to smoke, what to drink, and what weight to be.[5] People can lose weight by eating less and exercising more. Recognizing that people choose their weight for reasons other than health (e.g. they also like to look good), we allow appearance (A) to enter the utility function. For simplicity, assume that the utility from food and drink consumption is represented

---

[3] Shogren (2005).   [4] Becker (1965).
[5] Chen et al. (2002); Chou et al. (2002).

by calorie intake (K), a common assumption.[6] Leisure is assumed to be time remaining after work, exercise, and meal preparation.

We now write the consumer's utility function as a general equation which specifies what factors influence utility without specifying an exact mathematical relationship:[7]

$$U = u(K, S, L, H, A, Z).$$

We next specify a health function, again as a general relationship describing which variables influence health. Health (H) is related to weight (W), other aspects of diet quality (D_Q), such as the intake of saturated fatty acids, which may have an impact on health independent of weight, smoking (S), medical treatment (M), exercise (E), which is taken to provide health benefits independent of its impact on weight, and other exogenous factors (O_H), which include genetic and socio-demographic factors. These factors include education, which affects one's knowledge and ability to combine health inputs to optimize the health function.[8] Write the health state as:

$$H = h(W, S, M, E, D_Q, O_H).$$

For now we abstract from dynamics and time. Dynamics would recognize that current health depends on past levels of weight, diet quality, smoking, and exercise.

Weight gain occurs when calorie intake exceeds calorie expenditure. Calorie expenditure depends on activity in the workplace, in travel (by car, foot, or bicycle) and at home for leisure and non-leisure exercise; on metabolic rate (the genetic component to overweight and obesity); and on weight. As we discussed in Chapter 1, there is a steady state weight associated with any level of calorie intake. Within the behavioral framework established here, exercise itself is *endogenous*, which means that it is determined by the interaction with the other variables of the model, since a person may choose to achieve any particular weight either by consuming a large number of calories and exercising a lot or by consuming a lower number of calories and exercising less. *Exogenous* variables—for example, genetic inclination toward obesity—are determined outside the model, i.e. they do not depend on others in the model.

One assumption to simplify the model is to treat physical activity at work as exogenous (that people do not choose jobs to control their weight). One can express these ideas as another general mathematical relationship to indicate which variables affect a person's weight:

$$W = w(K, E, O_W)$$

where O_W represents exogenous factors such as the level of physical activity at work and genetic predisposition. We divide calorie intake into three categories: calories from home-prepared foods (K_H), from prepared foods purchased for home consumption (K_P), and from meals eaten outside the home (K_O).

---

[6] See e.g. Cutler et al. (2003); Lakdawalla and Philipson (2002); Philipson and Posner (1999).

[7] The exact relationship would vary for every individual according to their preferences.

[8] Chen et al. (2002).

$$K = K_H + K_P + K_O.$$

The utility function is maximized subject to the health function, the weight function, the calorie identity, and a budget constraint in which time may be enjoyed as leisure, transformed into income at the prevailing wage rate, used for exercise or used to create household goods such as meals. Food, drink, cigarettes, health care, and other goods up to the level of income may be purchased at prevailing prices.

$$W_R[T - L - E - G] = P_{KH}K_H + P_{KP}K_P + P_{KO}K_O + P_{DQ}D_Q$$
$$+ P_S S + P_M M + P_Z Z$$

where W_R is the wage rate, T is total time available (24 hours per day), L is time spent in leisure activities, including sleeping, E is exercise time, and G is time spent producing household goods.

The consumer can choose income (the product on the left-hand side of the above equation). Income is the wage rate times the hours he chooses to work. Calorie intake, smoking, the level of medical treatment, weight, exercise, and health status are all chosen by the person to maximize utility. The variables outside his control are the wage rate (W_R) and the market prices of food and drink (P_{KH}, P_{KP}, P_{KO}), diet quality (P_{DQ}), smoking (P_S), medical treatment (P_M), and goods unrelated to health (P_Z). The consumer cannot control the levels of the exogenous variables (O_H and O_W). If medical treatment is provided by the state, it is also exogenous to the person. The effectiveness of medical treatment is determined by technological developments over which he has no control.

Consumers consider the uncontrollable elements of their environment when they make decisions. For example, uncontrollable factors include food prices, current salary, effectiveness of medical treatments, and genetic characteristics. The controllable decisions include food consumption, the allocation of time between work and leisure, and the allocation of leisure time between physically active leisure and, say, watching television.[9] The model helps us to predict better the direction of change in any of the controllable variables given a change in the uncontrollable factors. We can define the key trade-offs people make in food choices and to understand how we react to changes in relative prices and income. This model also suggests how to specify the empirical models which quantify how people respond to changes in economic circumstances.

[9] We recognize that simplifying assumptions are not always observed in reality: people cannot always choose exactly how many hours they work because jobs specify weekly hours and holiday entitlements; though overtime can be an option, one may choose to work part-time, or one may work longer hours than contracted to gain promotion in the future. Which shows that even the wage rate is not truly exogenous—and extensions of the model can 'endogenize' wages even more by viewing education and training as investment decisions taken to improve future earnings. In addition, people get pleasure from exercise and cooking; and it may be reasonable to argue that diet quality is, at least partially, determined by decisions of whether to make food from raw ingredients, buy purchased foods, or eat out, though it is possible to buy healthy prepared food from supermarkets and restaurants.

This is the rub. Economists and the biomedical community can differ on how to frame policy because they differ about what is a controllable and uncontrollable factor in obesity. Biomedical studies, for instance, use a mind–body dualism that sees mental and biochemical processes as separable. This view holds that the conceptual tools of chemistry and physics applied to the body suffice to explain observed associations between nutrition and human health outcomes. The possibility that nutrition choices are made conditional on health outcomes is not modeled. Instead, epidemiological approaches treat endogenous dietary choices as uncontrollable. This view is exemplified in an editorial statement in a prestigious medical journal: 'Research on exogenous causes of hypertension has focused on diet, physical activity, and psychological factors' (Lenfant 1996). The implication is that biomedicine studies focus on the sources of hypertension without feeling impelled to explain the economics at work in dietary choices and exercise.

But, as documented by the economist Robert Fogel in his 1993 Nobel Prize speech, improvements in human health and lifespan over the last century have increased labor productivity and economic growth. These health improvements were credited to better nutrition and to an improved ability of people to transform nutrition information into better health states. At the same time, Fogel called for joint use of biomedical and economic techniques of analysis so that the consequences of better nutrition for human well-being can be examined in more depth. The combined techniques would yield insight otherwise unobtainable when relying on one of the disciplines alone. Fogel's call for combined techniques has rarely been followed, either in the biomedicine or in the health economics literatures.

Empirical estimates that maintain a separation of economic and biomedical factors are, in statistical terms, biased and inconsistent. The economics literature in the area of health and nutrition has focused on the willingness of the public to select eating habits consistent with the biomedical findings.[10] By accepting the causal implications of the biomedical model, the economics literature has revealed a curious inconsistency. A person is viewed as caring about his health state and having the discretion to affect health via choices of what he eats. But the knowledge base from the biomedical research does not address the role of those endogenous nutrition choices on health outcomes. Nutrition studies showing how health inputs (nutrients, exercise, medicines, visits to physicians, etc.) are

---

[10] Behrman and Wolfe (1989); Kenkel (1991); Variyam et al. (1999).

affected by people's choices are few; these studies are found in the economics literature.[11]

Those few attempts in biomedicine to introduce behavioral considerations do not model how individuals' decisions about what they eat depend upon prices and income. The estimated health response to a price-induced change in any one nutrient is an amalgam of the health responses to changes in consumption of all health inputs induced by the original price change. Though, in principle, laboratory studies of the health consequences of nutrient intake can eliminate the endogeneity issue through experimental controls, extrapolations of laboratory results in the form of dietary recommendations may prove misleading. Nutrient choices, which are constrained by the experimental design, may not reflect the unconstrained choices of consumers. Consequently, recommended changes in the consumption of one nutrient may induce people to alter their consumption of other health inputs as well. The extent to which they choose to do so depends on factors such as preferences, wages, prices, and income.[12] The everyday health outcomes of following the recommendation may differ from the laboratory result. Box 2.2 provides a good example, related not to obesity but nutrient demand and health.

Box 2.2. Case study: Sodium, blood pressure, and economics: a bio-behavioral model

As discussed above, economic theory sees food choice and health to be jointly determined (in statistical terms they are endogenous) and in this case study we present empirical evidence on why a presumption of independence (exogeneity) between biomedical conditions and economic circumstances can lead to biased predictions about food consumption and health decisions. We present the results of a study by Chen et al. (2002). They explore how individual choices on nutrient intake, exercise, and use of medication are influenced by economic circumstances, such as food prices, wages, and non-labor income. Accounting for the joint determination of food choice and health and the role of economic factors leads to differences in findings compared to epidemiological studies: for example, the impact of sodium on blood pressure changes from positive to negative (and statistically significant). Nearly 50 million Americans have high blood pressure, which increases risk of heart attack, stroke, and renal failure. Chen et al. (2002) estimate the direction and intensity of blood pressure response to changes in personal diet, exercise, and medication, assuming that people can choose these health inputs, and that economic variables such as wages, food prices, and income influence these choices.

---

[11] e.g. Behrman and Deolalikar (1988); Pitt and Rosenzweig (1986); Strauss (1986).
[12] Shogren and Crocker (1999).

As explained in Box 2.1, a person combines time, human capital, and purchased goods to produce utility from health, leisure, and other commodities. A person's health condition is also determined by his consumption of different nutrients, time spent exercising, the 'level' of medication consumed, and other observable personal and environmental attributes like education and gender. There are also fundamental biomedical attributes such as genetic and health endowments.

Two empirical models were constructed, an epidemiological model relating blood pressure to nutrient intake but without economic behavioral variables (the *Epi-only model*); and the *economic model* based on utility maximization, which includes wealth, wages, the total time that can be allocated to leisure, work, or exercise, shadow prices for nutrients (i.e. the price of one nutrient relative to another), and the price of medication.

In this *economic model*, a person's level of health is endogenous to his choices. Empirical specifications guided by this *structural model* allow biological and economic contributions to health states to be distinguished.

Chen et al. (2002) consider a sample of about 2,000 people who participated in the second cycle of the US National Health and Nutrition Examination Survey (NHANES II) between February 1976 and April 1978. NHANES II examined its participants' blood pressures and used questionnaires to acquire information on their medical histories, food consumption in the non-holiday weekday preceding the day of the blood pressure examination, and demographics. NHANES is a comprehensive data set on health and nutrition.

NHANES II translated food consumption information into daily intakes of seventeen nutrients. The work includes nine of the nutrients that the biomedical literature said could alter blood pressure. These nutrients are: fat, calcium, potassium, sodium, vitamin C, cholesterol, riboflavin, fatty acid balance, and oleic acid.

NHANES II also incorporates a number of indicators of participants' exogenous health endowments, including age in years (*age*), income (*income*), gender (*male*), education in years (*education*), and number of persons in the household (*hhold size*).

The first column of Table 2.1 reports the estimates of the benchmark epidemiological (epi-only) model. All statistically significant variables in the first column of the table have signs conforming to findings common in the biomedical literature. When the signs differ from those predicted by the biomedical literature, their associated coefficients fall well short of statistical significance.

The results in the second column show why accounting for economic circumstances matters. Now, for example, the result for calcium is that controlling for endogeneity in an economic context makes the nutrient appear to be about twenty-five times more effective in reducing blood pressure than does the estimate assuming calcium intake is exogenous in an epidemiological model. When endogenous activity choices are accounted for in the estimation, recreational exercise becomes fourteen times more effective at reducing systolic blood pressure, while taking medicine is associated with increased blood pressure.

The findings of epidemiological and laboratory studies of sodium intake impacts on blood pressure are mixed.[13] The table reproduces this ambiguity, a continuing source of controversy in the medical profession.[14] Sodium intake has no appreciable

---

[13] Midgley et al. (1996).
[14] Greenland (2001) and references therein.

impact on blood pressure when it is treated as exogenous in the epi-only model. But treating sodium intake as endogenous in the second column results in a negative and significant estimated impact on blood pressure: increased sodium intake lowers blood pressure. The open question to which we can provide a speculative response is why sodium intake has a negative effect on blood pressure. The challenge with changing salt in the diet is that other things change too. The estimated demand system reflects these multifaceted adjustments; a person uses salt to complement (read: 'spice up') what might otherwise seem a bland vegetable diet of, say, cooked broccoli and cauliflower. We observe that high sodium intake is associated with higher intake of vegetables and lower intake of other foods. This suggests that the effect of reduced salt intake is reduced vegetable intake and increased intake of other foods and nutrients, and the combined effect is to raise blood pressure despite sodium intake falling.

Table 2.1. Systolic blood pressure functions (N = 1982)

Intercept	Benchmark epi-only model	Two-stage structural economic model
Nutrient choices		
ln(fat)	−	+
ln(calcium)	− ***	− ***
ln(sodium)	+	− ***
ln(potassium)	+	+
ln(cholesterol)	−	− ***
ln(vitamin C)	+	+
ln(riboflavin)	+	+ ***
ln(fatty acids)	+ **	+ *
ln(oleic acids)	−	− **
Activity choices		
exercise	− **	− ***
medicine	+ **	+ ***
Demographics		
ln(age)	− ***	−
$[ln(age)]^2$	+ ***	+
male	+ ***	+ ***
ln(education)	− ***	+

Dependent variable: natural logarithm of systolic blood pressure.

* Significance at the .1 level. ** Significance at the .05 level. *** Significance at the .01 level.

The findings reinforce the idea that economic choices and health status are a two-way street: our choices affect our health, our health affects our choices. This seems obvious, and yet it is usually overlooked. A better understanding of how economic behavior and biology interact can lead to better health policy.

In relation to obesity, what insight do we gain from our benchmark model? First, the model captures the fundamental trade-off between eating for survival and overeating for pleasure. Assume a person has an ideal weight for health and appearance. Any deviations from this ideal—above or below—will reduce utility. If the person is below his ideal weight, he gains utility from eating more—both from the intrinsic pleasure and from weight gain. If he is above his ideal weight, he trades off the gains from eating against the losses in being heavier. People can choose to be somewhat heavier than their ideal: up to a certain point the gain in utility from eating more today exceeds the loss from being heavier in the future. But beyond a point, the losses in utility from weighing more exceed the gains from eating more. Each person's optimal weight depends on his own preferences for eating and drinking, income, the relative prices of goods and services, the importance he attaches to appearance and future health, and his genetic predisposition to gain weight. The main point from an economics perspective is that it can be *rational* to *choose* to be overweight.

We again emphasize this point: in our model of demand in which informed consumers make rational decisions, market failure is not the issue. Consumers weigh the personal costs when deciding whether to be overweight, including costs associated with the discomfort (or worse) of obesity-related ill health and medical expenses and lost earnings they themselves bear. This has led economists to call for the privatization of health systems. They argue that if people had to consider all the costs of their actions (including the full costs of medical treatment presently borne by society) they would take fewer risks; but if they want to take risks, they should be entitled to, provided they bear the consequences. In reality, political decisions in developed countries imply that the state bears health care costs and loss of earnings from illness. The political system has created a policy that leads to market failure: because people do not bear all of the costs of their actions, they impose costs on others (i.e. taxpayers). This is a rationale for policy intervention to prevent people from choosing to be overweight.

Second, the benchmark model helps economists to understand better how changes in economic circumstances (e.g. relative prices, technology) affect how people revise their choices in health care and consumption of food, and this can lead to a number of empirically testable hypotheses. Note that the first sets of hypotheses are all outcomes of our model of rational behavior in a well-functioning market; they do not rely on market failure. When it is available, we provide empirical evidence relating to the hypotheses.

Hypothesis 1. Lower food prices have increased the demand for food, leading to greater obesity.

Hypothesis 1A. Within the food group, prices have fallen more sharply for less healthy, more energy-dense food products such as processed and fast foods, resulting in their increased consumption.

A commonsense prediction coming from the economic model is that people respond to a change in relative prices by consuming more of the cheaper good and less of the expensive one. As agricultural and food technology has advanced, producers have become more productive—supplying more food at lower cost, translating into lower food prices. *Real prices* for food in Europe, the UK, and the US have fallen since 1960 (see Figure 2.1). Real prices measure how the price of food changes relative to the price of all goods, in this case using the year 2000 as a benchmark. Prices are expressed as real indices: they are divided by the overall consumer price index and refer to a given year, so the lines in Figure 2.1 show how prices evolved compared to the mean trend for all consumer goods. Consider the UK. In the UK food prices rose fourfold from 1975 to 2006. But since the prices for all goods and services rose by even more (fivefold), this means that food was cheaper in *real* terms by around 20% in 2006.

The fall in real prices during the 1980s matches up with the emergence of the obesity 'epidemic'. Did this decline in real food prices lead to increased obesity rates? This explanation loses support when one considers

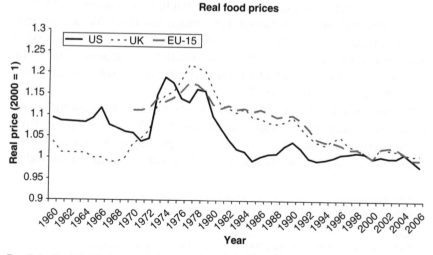

Real food prices

FIG. 2.1. Real food prices in the US, UK, and Europe, 1960–2006
Source: Our processing on data from Thomson Datastream (2007).

Elasticity

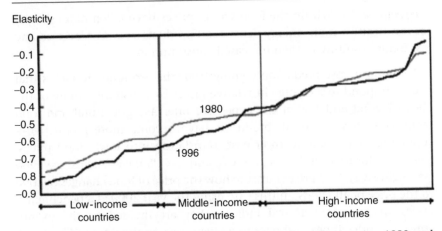

FIG. 2.2. Own-price elasticity for food in a cross-section of countries, 1980 and 1996

Source: 1996 data are Economic Research Service/United States Department of Agriculture estimates based on International Comparison Project data; 1980 data are from Theil et al. (1989), reproduced from Regmi et al. (2001).

the *price elasticity* of demand for food, which gives the percentage change in demand brought about by a 1% change in the price. Figure 2.2 shows the overall food demand elasticity in rich countries is close to zero—this means people are not very responsive to a change in real prices. Falling prices for food have a modest impact on overall food consumption,[15] an elasticity of −0.1 indicating that the 20% fall in food prices would lead to consumption increasing by around 2%, much less than calorie consumption has increased in developed countries (see Table 1.3). In the middle income countries, however, the price elasticity is around −0.5. This means a reduction in price of 20% would increase consumption by 10%, a significant growth in calorie intake.[16]

We now turn to look in more detail at price movements for individual foods and non-foods as shown in Figure 2.3. This figure shows three pairs of graphs. In the top line, the first graph shows the decline in real commodity prices (deflated by the IMF world consumer price index)

---

[15] While one might argue that the rise in calories might be due to an increase in energy density, it has been shown in Chapter 1 that most diets in developed countries have become closer to the WHO recommendations over time, which means a reduction in energy density.

[16] Since we wrote this book, attention has turned dramatically to the crisis of rising food prices. We won't speculate whether this will become a long-term reversal of the downward food price trend, but note that higher food prices will reduce calorie consumption, particularly in poorer countries.

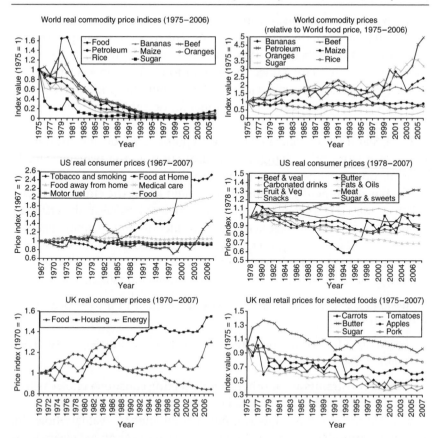

Fig. 2.3. Real price trends

Sources: Commodity prices from IMF International Financial Statistics (2007); US prices from Thomson Datastream; UK retail prices from UK Office for National Statistics (2007).

between 1975 and 2006. This figure illustrates the decrease in prices of raw food over time. The parallel graph on the right provides details on selected commodities (deflated by the average raw-food price) and suggests that fruit prices (bananas and oranges) decreased less than prices for beef, rice, maize, and sugar. These are raw-commodity prices, however; what matters to consumers is retail prices.

The middle two graphs show the evolution of consumer price indices in the US. Between 1967 and 2007 the prices of food consumed at home and out of the home decreased in real terms, but far less than petrol or tobacco. On the right-hand side, the relative prices of selected foods are illustrated. We see evidence that fruit and vegetables became relatively more expensive than sugar, carbonated drinks, and fats and oils, whose prices fell more than those for other foods. The bottom two graphs provide evidence for the UK between 1970 and 2007. Again, food prices decreased in real terms, but relative price changes for food items are less straightforward. Sugar prices became relatively lower, but the prices of fruit and vegetables like apples, carrots, and tomatoes decreased and butter prices increased.

The US and UK evidence related to hypothesis 1A on substitution induced by relative price changes is not clear-cut from the available data. In general, price changes in the US in particular have favored unhealthier foods, but the difficulty in being more certain about the effect of prices is missing data on relative price changes of processed versus fresh versus fast foods. If, as has been suggested, mass production and technological advances in food processing and fast foods has lowered their prices relative to unprocessed food and full-service restaurants, this would encourage consumption of processed and fast foods (see Chou et al. 2002).

Hypothesis 2. Rising incomes increase the demand for food (leading to greater obesity).

Hypothesis 2A. Income inequality in developed countries is associated with larger obesity rates.

Income constraints are another factor affecting consumer choice within the household production model. Over the last three decades, average per capita real income has increased, but it is difficult to evaluate how this may have impacted on calorie intakes and weight. At an aggregate level, one can merge FAO data on calorie availability with OECD information on aggregated food prices and gross domestic product. The merged data set provides information on twenty-four OECD countries over the period 1990–2002. After allowing for country-specific differences and accounting for endogeneity, a modeling exercise[17] returns an income elasticity of calorie demand for developed countries of 0.14, which means that a 1% increase in real per capita income translates into a 0.14% increase in calorie availability.

On average over this period, economic growth for these countries was around 2% per year, while mean calorie availability was 3,350 calories. This translates into a 4% increase in calories over the whole period 1990–2002, i.e. about 130 extra calories. Evidence of an income effect on

---

[17] The model is actually a panel simultaneous equation model with fixed effects; see Mazzocchi and Traill (2007).

obesity rates is rejected by Cutler et al. (2003) and others.[18] These studies have examined household data and found an inverse association between income and obesity. Since other health inputs like exercise increase with higher incomes, their results are compatible with consumer choices in which people take countermeasures for the increased calorie intake. On balance we reject hypothesis 2 and conclude that there is little evidence of a relationship between incomes and calorie intake and obesity in developed countries. But, as we discussed in Chapter 1, in less developed countries income growth can be an important force for increased calorie intake and obesity.

Empirical evidence on hypothesis 2A is not unequivocal. There are several studies in the public health literature that point to income inequalities as a determinant of obesity in developed countries,[19] because of lower dietary quality and leisure physical activity of poor households.[20] While a negative relationship between BMI and household income is a common result,[21] there are many confounding factors, especially race and gender, as this inverse relationship holds for women, but not necessarily for men.[22] While a negative relationship is found between income and energy intakes which could be consistent with hypothesis 2A[23] and the previous rejection of hypothesis 2, things are less clear on the energy expenditure side. Inconsistencies seem to depend on the role of income in determining different levels of physical activity. Income acts on physical activity in two directions, as higher incomes are associated with more sedentary jobs, but also with higher leisure time physical activity,[24] which explains why the final outcome in terms of BMI is not certain.

Hypothesis 3. The time cost of food preparation has fallen, resulting in people consuming more ready-prepared foods and meals outside the home. Because these foods tend to be more energy-dense, this has encouraged higher calorie intake.

The household production function model recognizes that time and money are constraints to households. As people respond to price changes by switching from high-priced to low-priced goods, similarly they respond to changes in the relative time cost by switching from high to low time cost activities. Such switching activity is greatest between close substitutes.

---

[18] See e.g. Silberberg (1985); Subramanian and Deaton (1996); Adelaja et al. (1997).
[19] See e.g. Pickett et al. (2005).
[20] Drewnowski and Specter (2004).
[21] See also Chou et al. (2004).
[22] See Chang and Lauderdale (2005) and references therein.
[23] See e.g. Chesher (1997).
[24] Lakdawalla and Philipson (2002).

While some people may enjoy food preparation, others find the daily duty of food preparation a drudge. Time spent preparing food cannot be spent on leisure activities, or working to earn more money, which could be spent on other things. Technological advances have created new and cheaper prepared food; developments in home technology have reduced the cost of refrigerator, freezer, and microwave so that they are now ubiquitous in developed countries and common in developing countries among middle-income consumers.

Cutler et al. (2003) refer to this as *mass preparation* in centralized factories replacing individual preparation in the home. The mass preparation of food has followed the similar, much earlier, revolution in mass production of other manufactured goods. Cutler et al. demonstrate their argument with respect to the humble potato chip (or French fry), once a rare treat in the home owing to the time cost of peeling, slicing, and cooking potatoes into chips—people instead ate their potatoes boiled or baked. Now they buy their chips frozen and oven-ready, preparation time is near zero, resulting in an increase in the share of potatoes consumed as chips: in 1970, 31% of potatoes in America were purchased frozen, but by 1995 this proportion had increased to 54% and at the same time overall potato consumption had increased by 30%.

In general, the results of this process of technological change have been dramatic increases in the range of prepared foods available to households and improvements in quality so that they are as good as you could produce by slaving over a hot stove for several hours—cakes, salted snacks, ready meals, and prepared fruit and vegetables are all at our fingertips. As Cutler et al. (2003) say, labor in the home has been replaced by labor in the factory and supermarket; the average household time spent preparing food and clearing up after meals has halved since the mid-1960s.

What has this to do with obesity? If a piece of cake with the afternoon tea or coffee 'costs' a couple of hours' mixing and baking, one might think twice about it. Instead, if one can open the cupboard, the time cost involved is minimal and temptation is higher. There is extra shopping, which is easier today since people can drive to supermarkets; even in middle-income developing countries supermarkets are where people shop.[25] Consumers respond by eating more manufactured foods and doing so more frequently. Cutler et al. (2003) examined data from the US Continuing Survey of Food Intake in 1977–8 and 1994–6. They found that increased snacking explained nearly all Americans' increased calorie intake over this period.[26]

[25] Reardon and Berdegue (2002); Reardon et al. (2003); Traill (2006) and references therein.
[26] Though this finding is not supported in a survey of snacking and weight gain among schoolchildren (Field et al. 2004).

Greater use of convenience foods also results from households having less leisure time available as the number of working married women has increased over the years. In the Anglophone countries of Australia, Canada, the US, and the UK, female labor force participation averaged 57% in 1980 and grew to 67% by the end of the 1990s.[27]

Hypothesis 4A. Improvements in medical technology that reduce the health risks of obesity encourage people to increase their weight.

Suppose there is a technological advance in medical treatment, e.g. better screening and medicine for hypertension. A person can increase their utility by: (i) consuming unchanged levels of other variables in the health function (Box 2.1) such as smoking, eating, and alcohol, thereby gaining much improved health, or (ii) compensating for the health advantages of the new technology by indulging in higher levels of health-reducing activities like smoking, eating, and drinking. In other words, better medical technology allows people to choose to weigh more given the lower risks associated with obesity. The response to the new technology depends on the relative importance of health and appearance in the utility function. If appearance is the overriding factor, improvements in medical technology will have little impact. But if health is important, the changes may be significant.

Hypothesis 4B. Reductions in smoking reduce smoking-related health risks, thereby enabling people to take other health risks, including those associated with obesity.

This is the same logic as for the impact of improvements in health technology. Social norms have changed, so the utility derived from smoking has fallen. If you smoke less, your health improves, but, as above, there is a possible rebound effect: you can now engage in other risky activities like putting on weight by eating more (or exercising less). In this framework, a behavioral explanation exists for the observed negative correlation between smoking and weight.[28] The medical literature[29] has attributed this correlation to increased caloric intake and decreased metabolic rate when giving up smoking.[30] While these reasons may be valid, the economic perspective adds a behavioral explanation. The example mirrors similar

---

[27] De Laat and Sevilla Sanz (2006).

[28] See e.g. Chou et al. (2002); Gruber and Frakes (2006); Picone and Sloan (2003); Loureiro and Nayga (2005).

[29] See Filozof et al. (2004).

[30] See e.g. Flegal et al. (1995); Rodu et al. (2004).

evidence with respect to other risky behavior; for example, evidence suggesting that safer cars and the compulsory wearing of seatbelts have encouraged motorists to choose to drive faster.

Let us summarize this section before moving on to extend the model in a couple of important ways.

- Markets can fail in three important ways:
  1. consumption creates externalities—costs borne by others than the person consuming the good;
  2. people may not be perfectly informed; and
  3. there may be market power in the industry, so prices charged by firms do not reflect the cost of the resources used in production.

- A comprehensive model of the consumer decision-making process shows that obesity does not necessarily imply market failure provided people account for the costs of their overindulgence, including related medical expenses and lost productivity. In reality, in developed countries these costs are borne by society at large, so society has created a system where obesity can be seen as a market failure.

- Regardless of whether obesity is a market failure, the household production model generates hypotheses which can shed light on the emergence of the obesity epidemic and make predictions about future change. First, relative prices are important predictors of consumption; falling real food prices over the past twenty years and the falling price of processed and fast foods relative to unprocessed foods are likely important drivers of increased calorie intake. Second, relative time costs of goods can affect their consumption; in the case of food, technological advances permitting mass production of processed foods and meals away from home combined with less total time available to households is likely the key factor to have driven consumption of processed foods and meals outside the home. Third, people substitute risks; advances in medical technology and the reduced prevalence of smoking may have encouraged people to risk being more overweight.

Model Extension

We now consider extensions to the economic model which are useful in understanding and evaluating consumer behavior on healthy eating. We continue to assume, for the moment, that consumers make informed choices.

TIME PREFERENCE

The household production model has focused on decisions in one time period. We now consider how time affects choice. We highlight three key temporal issues for obesity: two biological and one behavioral. First, current weight is affected by current calorie intake and exercise, and by past intake and expenditure of calories and past energy expenditure. Second, the effects of excess weight on health occur with substantial time lags. Third, the important behavioral relationships occur because people discount the future. A good available now is valued more highly than the same good promised in, say, ten years' time, and, in the same way, a 'bad', such as poor health, promised for ten years' time is not as bad as it would be coming today. This means that people obtain greater utility from $100 today than from $100 in ten years' time. This *discounting* idea should be built into the utility function, recognizing that utility from present consumption of food and drink is immediate, as is disutility from exercising, whereas utility gains from improved health are years away.[31] By contrast, the impact on appearance of excess calorie intake, if not immediate, is much closer in time and so should be accorded greater weight in people's decision making.

This implies that how a factor affects a person's utility depends on three things: the importance attached to the factor (e.g. health), the length of the lag between an action and its consequences (eating too much leading to putting on weight leading to adverse health consequences), and the rate at which a person discounts the future. Two people with identical propensities to put on weight and identical preferences for eating and drinking, health, appearance, leisure, and so forth may make different choices because they have different time preferences—the 'myopic' one who lives for today (who, in economists' terminology, has a high discount rate or high rate of time preference) emphasizes current consumption and so is more likely to be overweight than her long-sighted, 'sensible' neighbor who is prepared to forgo pleasure today in favor of a better life in the future.

These ideas are straightforward and uncontroversial in principle, and rather difficult to use in practice because measuring people's individual time preferences remains challenging.[32] When evaluating the costs and benefits of a proposed public policy, economists discount the future using

---

[31] A comprehensive review of the economic literature on time preference and discounting can be found in Frederick et al. (2002).

[32] See Harrison et al. (2002).

a revealed time preference value from the market. For example, in appraising an investment that requires giving up something now for a larger future return, one can use the rate at which current consumption can be exchanged for future consumption in risk-free financial markets. If your local bank pays 5% p.a. on savings, but inflation reduces spending power by 2% p.a., the real rate of return is 3%. Without getting into a detailed discussion of financial economics, let us say this real rate of return of 3% p.a. is a market outcome (an 'equilibrium', as explained in the opening section of this chapter) arising from the interaction of millions of individuals' savings and borrowing decisions. These decisions can be thought of as a demand and supply process: the higher the rate of return, the more people are willing to save, the less they are prepared to borrow; the lower the rate of return, the converse. Only at the market equilibrium rate of interest are savings and borrowings equal, and in this sense they reflect society's time preference in the same way that the price of carrots reflects society's valuation of the worth of carrots. This real return on a risk-free investment has been used by economists and others in discounting the future. Typical values employed are 1.5% to 3.5% p.a.

Discounting, however, raises pertinent behavioral questions such as: Are people's time preferences for health the same as for money? How do time preferences vary across individuals in society and how are these related to demographics, education, income, social status, and age? Are individuals consistent in their time preferences as they get older? Do children have any concept of the future or must adults decide for them?

In relation to age, even if the discount rate is invariant over time, the existence of a time preference can explain why young people are less concerned about adverse health effects of overeating than older people. For a 20-year-old, the disutility from becoming, say, a diabetic at age 70, discounted at 3% p.a. is 23% $(=1/(1.03)^{50})$ of the disutility from the same condition today (48% if discounted at 1.5%). But for a 60-year-old, the disutility is 74% $(=1/(1.03)^{10})$ of the condition today. If health were the only concern, it would be rational for a young person to eat less healthily than an older person.[33] We do observe young people eating less fruit and vegetables and more snack foods than older people. For example, data from the UK National Diet and Nutrition Survey[34] shows that the

---

[33] Of course young people are more concerned with their appearance and this may counteract their discounting the health risks. Also we do not predict that young people would be more overweight than old people because there are so many other forces at work—not least, slowing metabolic rates during the ageing process.

[34] See Swan (2004).

percentage of energy from nutrients like saturated fats and carbohydrates is higher for the group aged 19–24 and declines as age increases, while intakes of vitamins follow the opposite path. Similar results can be found in Italy.[35] The percentage of Italians who consume one portion of fruit and vegetables per day or less is greater during youth (about 21% between 18 and 34) and declines at older ages (16% between 45 and 54, 13% above 60). NHANES data for the US[36] confirm that teenagers consume twice the saturated fat of those who are 40–59 years old.

Measuring individuals' discount rates is problematic, but economists have attempted to do so and have found the expected relationships between people's implied discount rate and smoking behavior,[37] college drinking,[38] and drug taking.[39] Such findings have been used to suggest that a person's indulgence in smoking, drinking and drug taking, and other time-related behavior may be used as proxy variables for the discount rate. For example, Huston and Finke (2003) use as proxies whether a person smokes, whether he or she takes regular exercise, and his or her level of education (also viewed as an investment which involves forgoing current income and consumption for higher future levels) to explain healthy eating in the US, and the signs of the variables are consistent with the discounting hypothesis. Smokers, non-exercisers, and the poorly educated are presumed to discount the future more heavily as revealed by their reluctance to forgo current pleasures, and they are also found to eat less healthily. The trouble with using these proxies is that there may be other reasons than time preference why people smoke, exercise, or are educated. This proxy approach attributes all of the causal relationship to time preference.

Komlos et al. (2004) examine the relationship between the net domestic saving rate and the obesity rate in a selection of countries. The lower the rate of savings, the lower the value people place on the future relative to the present—i.e. the higher the discount rate. While their research is still exploratory, they find the data are consistent with a negative relationship between the two variables; the less people care about the future, the more obese they are. They move a step further, hypothesizing that the recent obesity trends may be explained by an increase in the discount rate of the

[35] Italian Multi-Purpose Survey, *Indagine multiscopo sulle famiglie: Aspetti della vita quotidiana*, <http://www.istat.it/dati/catalogo/20071106_00/>.
[36] Ervin et al. (2004).
[37] Fuchs (1982).
[38] Vuchinich and Simpson (1999).
[39] Bretteville-Jensen (1999).

population as a whole—implying that people live for the present more than they used to in decades past.

Smith et al. (2005) provide an empirical test of the hypothesis advanced by Komlos et al., using US nationally representative panel data from the National Longitudinal Survey of Youth over the period 1979–89 and again considering data on saving and withdrawing money over time as a proxy for time preference. After accounting for income, age, and ethnicity, they find evidence of a higher BMI for those who have not increased their saving over time, especially men.

Time preference studies have been carried out to explore rising obesity rates in Europe, too. For example, Borghans and Golsteyn (2006) look at the relation between discounting rates and BMI in the Netherlands, exploring the relationship both in cross-section terms and over time. Their findings confirm the role of time discounting in affecting obesity. Overall, however, the empirical evidence is still weak. A concern with all these studies is that other factors may have generated changes in saving levels.[40]

In concluding this section, we reiterate that while more research is needed on the influence of time preference on obesity rates, discounting is not a market failure but a rational way of balancing and trading off distant and proximate consumption.

SELF-CONTROL, ADDICTION, AND RELATED EXPLANATIONS

We have so far credited our rational consumer with great foresight and consistency to be able to make utility-maximizing decisions involving trade-offs between consumption choices years apart. But we know in reality we are not always consistent. We know something is bad for us, and by tomorrow we will regret doing it, but we are unable to resist the temptation of immediate gratification. We tell ourselves when we overindulge in cream cakes, chocolate, and ice cream today that we can always go on a diet tomorrow.[41] Circumstantial evidence exists to suggest that lack of self-control contributes to the obesity epidemic. The largest increase in weight in the United States is in the upper tail of the BMI probability distribution:[42] those who are already overweight or obese have become even more overweight or obese at a rate faster than the rest of the population. Lack of self-control in this group, alongside greater

---

[40] Zhang and Rashad (2008).
[41] Cutler et al. (2003).
[42] Cutler et al. (2003); McCormick and Stone (2007).

availability of energy-dense snack foods, greater time pressure, falling prices, and rising incomes, is a credible explanation.[43]

Economists have modeled this lack of self-control (or behavioral failure, as it is sometimes known) in a utility maximization framework by assuming that people's discount rate declines as the time horizon increases.[44] This implies that, while we care a lot about having to delay consumption from this year to next year, say, or from today until tomorrow when temptation is put in front of us, we are less concerned about delaying consumption from, say, ten years to eleven years in the future or from ten days until eleven days in the future. The finding of the modeling exercise is that people who suffer from lack of self-control do not make a rational choice which maximizes their overall lifetime welfare (from eating and their health), and their utility can be increased by their not being allowed to indulge in short-sighted behavior, for example by removing snack vending machines from schools and universities.[45] This is an unusual example where economists may accept that weight gain is not a personal utility-maximizing decision, though liberals and conservatives alike may find the prescription that the state should intervene to control people's behavior when no one else is harmed by their actions as taking the 'nanny state' a step too far.

Now consider the economics of addiction. Addiction is related to self-control but technically different from the economist's perspective. The open question is whether people can become addicted to food in the same way as they can become addicted to alcohol, drugs, and jogging. A necessary (but not sufficient) condition for addiction to occur is that a person's present consumption increases their future consumption of the same good.[46] Becker and Murphy (1988) show that addiction can be rational in the sense that it represents lifetime utility-maximizing behavior, unlike absence of self-control.

For food, the rational addiction model can be extended to explain cycles of overeating and dieting;[47] and people who discount the future heavily are most likely to become addicted, but because addiction in this economic model is rational, individuals' welfare could not be increased by government action. Is there any evidence for addiction to food? Evidence

---

[43] Physical–metabolic explanations are also credible—people can be susceptible to weight gain.

[44] The model is referred to as based on hyperbolic discounting; Frederick et al. (2002).

[45] Zhang and Rashad (2008).

[46] Becker and Murphy (1988).

[47] Levy (2002).

suggests that people can be addicted to food. The empirical work of Cutler et al. (2003) shows that increases in calorie intake in America come from carbohydrates, which scientific evidence suggests, especially sugar, may be addictive.[48]

Not even economists argue that all addiction is rational, so, as with self-control, the issue arises, first, whether people can become addicted to food, and, if so, whether it is a state role to intervene, as it does with drugs (by making them illegal) or tobacco and alcohol (by taxing them). The question of whether food addiction exists is an important one for future research by economists and natural scientists.

We conclude this section on discounting by asking whether the idea contributes to understanding observed changes in obesity over time or differences between social groups or countries. Theory and evidence provide no strong reason to suggest it does. Do people live for the present more than they used to (so care more about the pleasure of eating now than about adverse future health consequences)? There is no empirical evidence to support this view. Do cultural differences between countries explain the behavior? For example, the Japanese take a longer-term perspective on life than Anglo-Saxons. But again insufficient data exist to test empirically a relationship between time preference and obesity. One may also argue, without empirical evidence, that it is a working-class characteristic to live for the present while the middle classes think only of the future; and make an association with the fact that the working classes are more obese than the middle classes. Discounting is a plausible partial explanation for the differences in obesity levels we observe in the real world, between countries and social classes, but is unlikely to be the full story.

RISK AVERSION

Relationships between diet and health are probabilistic rather than known and deterministic. People behave differently under risky situations either because they attach different probabilities to the outcome or because they respond differently to risk: people differ in their aversion to risk. Attaching different probabilities may result from imperfect information, which may be associated with level of education, or from different abilities to control risks through private actions. Different assessments of risks associated with the same activity may be rational; for example, someone with parents

---

[48] The rational addiction hypothesis in relation to obesity is explored in Richards and Patterson (2006).

who are obese, heavy smokers, and drinkers but live to an old age may conclude that they have inherited 'good' genes and are less at risk of premature death from obesity than the average person.

Given a subjective probability of a risky event, the economist's approach is to assume that people maximize their expected utility. If eating a food can generate two outcomes, staying healthy and becoming sick, the expected utility can be expressed as a weighted average of the utilities of being healthy and sick, in which the weights are the subjective probabilities of being healthy and sick. These probabilities are affected by the choices people make about diet and exercise.

A *risk averse* person takes a payoff given with certainty over a fair bet with the same expected value of payoff (e.g. they prefer a certain €100 to a gamble with 50% chance of winning €200 and 50% chance of winning nothing). A person is said to be *risk loving* if they prefer the bet to the certain payoff and *risk neutral* if they are indifferent. We should observe a risk averse person taking fewer risks with their health than a risk loving person.

As with time preference, a measure of risk aversion determined by propensity to gamble for money need not necessarily carry forward to behavior about health. People do not necessarily behave in a consistent manner with respect to different types of risk, say financial and recreational. Weber et al. (2002), for example, developed separate scales to measure and predict individuals' behavior with respect to each of financial risks, health and safety risks, recreational risks, ethical risks, and social risks.

While studies exist on the relation between smoking and risk attitudes, the literature on overeating or obesity is not as rich. Among recent efforts, an interesting study is the one by Anderson and Mellor (2007). Based on experimental data, they relate a range of health behaviors to an individual index for risk aversion based on lottery choice. After controlling for various demographic and ethnic variables, they find a significant negative association between risk aversion and being overweight or obese, a relation which emerges as stronger than for smoking, binge drinking, speeding, or driving without wearing seatbelts.

Finally, as we said with respect to time preference, although risk aversion may contribute to explaining differences among individuals—or even social groups or countries—it cannot explain changes in the level of obesity over the past twenty or so years unless we believe people have become less risk averse over time. From an economist's perspective, people have different attitudes to risk; their rational behavior in risky situations is therefore different, but no one can say their preferences or behavior are 'right' or 'wrong'. They have nothing to do with market failure.

Conclusion

In this section, we have discussed how economics adds insight into how people make choices over food, health, and obesity. Economics puts a spotlight on the key trade-offs people confront; and how these trade-offs are affected by the circumstances they can control and those they cannot. The economist's role is to help to identify how relative prices, relative incomes, time constraints, discounting, and risk aversion affect a person's choices of what to consume, where, and how much, and also health status. Once we recognize the two-way behavioral relationship between how incomes affect health and how health affects incomes, we can better understand and target cost-effective policies aimed at improving overall health within a nation.

The economics of the demand side of obesity assumes that people behave with purpose, and this behavior does not necessarily correspond to the healthiest one. An economist's conclusion about what policies work and why can differ from the standard expectations based on purely natural science information. For instance, an economist would say that people might willingly gain weight because modern medical progress has reduced their overall health risks. An economist might also argue that people have a risk-taking portfolio; people who quit smoking to reduce risk might rebalance the risk portfolio by increasing other risks, like those caused by overeating. From the economist's perspective, public intervention is necessary to correct consumer behavior if people's choices generate uncompensated externalities on other people, but if our choices are informed and free, we should be entitled to make unhealthy choices.

Market Exchange: Information

Our discussion of the consumer so far suggests that obese people have freely chosen to be obese; they have made fully informed decisions given the economic circumstances they face. They may still impose external costs on others through the health service but as individuals their decisions are rational. Fully informed decisions, as we have assumed so far, are based on *complete information*. Buyers understand all their options and they understand the consequences of their actions.

Complete information implies that the consumer understands: (1) the link between their dietary and lifestyle choices and obesity; (2) the link between obesity and its health consequences, including knowledge about the relative risks and the costs; and (3) how to weigh these risks and costs of alternative possible outcomes. Those people who understand this information are assumed to make purposeful decisions about their own health. These purposeful decisions lead to a socially efficient outcome. The main question we should address is whether it is reasonable to assume that consumers are adequately informed of the consequences of their decisions, and, if not, whether it influences their decisions in a significant or systematic way.

Nobody, not even a nutritionist, is perfectly informed about the composition of all the food they eat and the health consequences of each and every action. The more important issue is whether systematic biases make them more likely to consume unhealthy food (and too much of it), and whether this likelihood has changed over time. Another key issue is whether education is a limiting factor.

Economists have argued that a market economy is best characterized as an exchange system with incomplete or asymmetric information. With incomplete or asymmetric information, it is no longer guaranteed that individual choices will aggregate into an outcome that is socially optimal. Imperfect information simply means that people do not know the exact relationships between their diets and their health risks. Asymmetric information is a special case where one person in a transaction, usually the seller, has more information than the other, the buyer. A food manufacturer, for instance, knows more about the safety and nutritional quality of food than a busy shopper, or the chef of a restaurant has much better information on the ingredients and the quality of the foods he cooks than the customer.

Economists have long discussed the impact of asymmetric information on market exchange, triggered by an influential article, 'The Market for Lemons' by the Nobel Laureate George Akerlof (1970). His paper considers the market for secondhand cars, termed 'lemons' if defective. The seller knows the cars' deficiencies but the buyer does not. The buyer will only pay the price of the average quality car sold in the market; this causes the higher-quality car sellers to exit the market because they cannot get the higher price. This exiting process continues until eventually only the lemons remain in the market. The market collapses if quality cannot be determined and protected by inspection or warranty.

The implications underlying the lemon model go beyond used cars, including questions about the functioning of the healthy food market. When the quality of food is uncertain, two consequences emerge: (1) high-quality food may be driven out of the market as buyers cannot distinguish them from lower quality produced at lower cost; and (2) as the average quality falls, the expected quality also falls and ultimately the price falls— leading to a further decrease in food quality and so on. Eventually, the market collapses so only the lowest-quality food remains unsold. For the market to survive, a trust relationship or a reduction in uncertainty is needed, like guarantees for durables or brand names for frequently purchased goods. Interestingly, Akerlof does consider hamburger restaurant chains and notes that hamburger eaters outside their local area may prefer the known quality of the fast food chain to the unknown quality of a local restaurant, even though local restaurants may on average supply a better quality than the chain.

For food choices, numerous information imperfections exist. They include the misperception of the role of calories and portion sizes; confusion and uncertainty about weight-loss methods; conflicting information about nutrition–health relationships; and difficulties in using nutritional information (e.g. relating calories and nutrient content to serving sizes).[49] Philipson (2001), however, argues that information issues are unlikely to be a cause of increasing obesity rates, given the rising amount of communication on obesity and its health risks. In contrast, other studies argue that the problem is less related to how much information is provided than to its ability to meet people's specific information needs and processing abilities.[50] Processing contradictory information may be problematic.

Nutrition labeling is the typical method to reduce asymmetric information; labeling works by transferring knowledge about nutrients from producers to consumers. According to the US Food and Drug Administration (FDA), after the introduction of the Nutrition Labeling and Education Act in 1993, 59% of US consumers changed their food purchases and 6,500 reduced-fat products were introduced to the market.[51] Reducing the information asymmetry has benefited both consumers and producers of healthy foods, as the equilibrium quantity increased.

One can argue that if a high rate of obesity is a market failure caused by incomplete information which led people to underestimate the health risks of excess weight, once informed about the real risks, people would

[49] Seiders and Petty (2004) and references therein.   [50] Verbeke (2005).
[51] Figures reported in Gardner (2003), who notices that this has not prevented obesity rates from increasing.

choose to lose weight. But evidence on the relation between health knowledge and weight is mixed. A US study exploring the relationship between diet–health knowledge, schooling, and obesity[52] has shown that increased knowledge—measured through a set of questions within the Diet and Health Knowledge Survey—was associated with reduced obesity, after controlling for factors like income and age. An international study promoted by WHO which twice surveyed (with a ten-year span) about 35,000 individuals in twenty-six countries[53] also found an inverse relationship between knowledge and obesity, but only for females, not males. Other studies, however, have found little or no relationship between knowledge and weight or the desire to lose weight.[54] From an economic point of view, the idea that more information does not always induce people to lose weight is not surprising. On the contrary, this result is consistent with the view that people choose freely to take risks and substitute between unhealthy behaviors, when relative risks change. Education and information measures are not a generic panacea when there is no clear substantiation of an information 'problem'.

Furthermore, suppliers of healthy foods have incentives to provide verifiable information on the positive characteristics of their products. This information 'signal' allows producers to differentiate their product on the market, through health claims and other nutrition information. Signaling is a market solution to the imperfect information problem. The market develops mechanisms so that better-quality goods are signaled by the most informed party, since both suppliers and consumers have an incentive to ensure their distinction from 'bad' goods. A natural example of signaling is a label whose content, in the absence of regulation, suppliers are forced to substantiate by developing trust and a reputation for honesty through branding.

Until the mid-1980s the US FDA had discouraged private health claims. But this policy changed after the well-publicized *Kellogg's* case. The Kellogg Company, in collaboration with the National Cancer Institute, promoted the health benefits of high-fiber cereals in preventing cancer.[55] This case is illustrative of a potential market failure due to inadequate information provision driven by 'free riding' of rival firms. Kellogg had an incentive to produce information about the health benefits of fiber in breakfast cereals. Their incentive was mitigated, however, because competitors could free

[52] Nayga (2000).
[53] Molarius et al. (2000).
[54] Kan and Tsai (2004); Burns et al. (1987); Hankey et al. (2004).
[55] Calfee and Pappalardo (1991).

ride the general health claim without incurring the costs of advertising. While Kellogg's high-fiber cereals increased their sales at the expense of non-high-fiber cereals, competitors gained even more than Kellogg.[56]

When free riding is a risk, or firms are too small to undertake advertising, one potential solution is generic advertising. As there is no incentive for a single producer to bear the costs of communicating the attributes of a product, groups of interested parties may band together to share the costs and jointly promote the advertising campaign. The results are predictable.[57] Generic advertising benefits some groups of producers at the expense of others: a 'beggar-thy-neighbor' outcome[58] (if people respond by eating more apples, say, in response to an apple promotion campaign, it is likely to be at the expense of other fruit; apple growers win, other fruit growers lose), especially because there is little substitution between healthy and unhealthy foods, as health claims have a weak effect on disease risk perceptions and they do not affect product evaluation or purchase intentions.[59]

Awareness does not (necessarily) lead to a healthier lifestyle as evidenced by a second example: an experimental test of a nutrition shelf-labeling scheme by the Stop & Shop supermarket chain in cooperation with the FDA.[60] The study involved twenty-five stores in four states. In twelve of these stores, several actions were tested, including shelf tags augmented with nutrition information, booklets, and posters, while no action was implemented in the remaining thirteen stores, which constituted the control group. Compared to shops in the control group, consumers receiving the additional information decided both to eat more healthy goods in some labeled categories and to eat less of others. They did so presumably because the additional information allowed them to make a better-informed choice among healthy foods without necessarily leading them to substitute between healthy and unhealthy foods. Economic reasoning does not contradict these results: the Stop & Shop consumers faced a series of trade-offs in which health could be an important factor but not the only one.

Another issue arises in the economics of information: *transaction costs*. Transaction costs are those associated with making a decision. Labeling food products costs money; reading labels takes time. Both producers

[56] See results from Levy and Stokes (1987).
[57] See Alston et al. (2000, 2001); Boetel and Liu (2003) and references therein.
[58] Alston et al. (2001).
[59] Garretson and Burton (2000).
[60] Teisl et al. (2001).

and consumers are constrained by the cost of information. Producers do not want to generate costly labels if rivals can free ride off their efforts or if consumers ignore the labels, or both. Consumers do not want to read labeling information if it does not improve their decision making sufficiently to compensate for the time spent. An informed purchase is more expensive than a less informed purchase because of these transaction costs. Transaction costs act as a barrier to information provision and use.

Advertising and Food Demand

Can people be persuaded to consume more by the provision of persuasive information? Significant sums of money are spent advertising food (see Table 2.2). This money is concentrated in the 'big five', pre-sugared breakfast cereals, soft drinks, confectionery, savory snacks, and fast food[61]—foods that would not be featured in healthy eating campaigns. Indeed, Lang and Heasman (2004) show that if you build a pyramid showing advertising expenditure on different classes of foods, it is the inverse of the US Department of Agriculture (USDA) healthy eating pyramid, which shows how much of different foods should be consumed in a healthy diet: there is little advertising of fresh fruit and vegetables (they remain unbranded), whole grain cereals, and the like.

It is a logical, though not necessarily correct, step to argue that the big companies that spend all this money are not dim-witted and would not spend it if advertising were ineffective.[62] We are reminded of the US retailer John Wanamaker's famous adage 'I know half my advertising is wasted. I just do not know which half.' He made that quip over a century ago, and computerized models have made advertising less of a lottery today. But it is still difficult to show that advertising has increased the consumption of one product at the expense of others (or in addition to others). For example, Zywicki et al. (2004) ask whether an advert for pizza encourages people to eat pizza for dinner whereas without the ad they would have selected boiled chicken and broccoli. Companies claim (as did the tobacco manufacturers) that their advertising is targeted at brand switching rather than expansion of the overall category. A review of

---

[61] Skinner et al. (2005).

[62] Advertising has other goals than to increase sales or market share. We recognized it may have a strategic role—to raise the costs of entry into an industry and thereby increase market power. It may also be used to enhance reputation, such as McDonald's response to the film *Super Size Me* (2004).

Table 2.2. Annual advertising budget for products or brands of food and beverages in the US, 2001

Product or brand	$ million
Beverages	
Coke, Diet Coke	224.0
Pepsi, Mountain Dew	226.0
Kool-Aid	15.9
Dasani bottled water	26.4
Aquafina bottled water	13.2
Candy	
Nestlé candy	65.0
Hershey's candy	55.0
M & M's candy	46.8
Snickers candy bars	46.4
Reese's candy	22.7
Savory Snacks	
Frito-Lay and Frito's chips/snacks	24.8
Dorito's tortilla chips	20.9
Ruffles potato chips	19.3
Bugles corn snacks	13.4
Fast Food Restaurants	
McDonald's	635.0
Burger King	298.0
KFC	206.5
Taco Bell	179.4
Pizza Hut	148.0

Source: Advertising Age, 24 June 2002.

studies looking into the impact of advertising on obesity is provided by Zywicki et al. (2004). They argue that if the 'advertising has caused the increase in obesity' hypothesis is to be borne out, certain criteria must be satisfied: people must be exposed to more advertising now than in the past—and if advertising is received via television, either people must be watching more television than in the past, there are more advertisements per hour, the adverts are more sophisticated and effective, or there has been a switch in advertising toward less healthy foods. According to Nielsen Media Research,[63] children (in America) spent less time watching television (in 1999) than they did a decade earlier, and more time in front of the computer—not free of advertising material, but 75% of all food manufacturers' advertising budgets and 95% of fast food advertising in the US is for TV adverts.[64]

Zywicki et al. also find no evidence of more advert time per hour of television. They argue that the now ubiquitous remote control has

[63] Zywicki et al. (2004).
[64] Story and French (2004).

enabled children to channel-hop away from commercials.[65] In a content analysis of children's advertising they found that the proportion of commercials devoted to food fell from 64% in the 1970s to 46% in the 1990s— a larger proportion of ads were devoted to toys, computer games, videos, and DVDs.

Given this evidence, it seems unlikely that increased exposure to advertising can explain the sharp rise in childhood obesity in the US in the past twenty years. This is not to deny the validity of studies that correlate obesity with hours of TV viewing. Watching television is a sedentary activity and it is tempting to take snacks and drinks while watching. But this would occur even if no food was advertised on television. Nor do these data say advertising has no effect on the food choices of children (or adults); rather they cannot explain the increase in obesity. A careful review of studies into the effects of advertising on children commissioned by the UK Food Standards Agency[66] found that food advertising does impact on the categories of food chosen and the brand.

Food manufacturers and retailers engage in activities classed as marketing but not advertising, including two-for-one and other price discounts and, contentiously, selling 'impulse purchase' goods like confectionery on eye-level displays and at checkouts in which the 'pester-power' of children is relied on to increase sales. We do not defend this practice, nor question its effectiveness, nor argue against measures taken to control it. We would, however, question whether such actions could be expected to make much difference to obesity given that they are far from new.

In summary, we have argued that:

(a) Imperfect information can exist in food and nutrition markets, which create a market failure and can justify government regulation.

(b) But it is unclear and perhaps unlikely that better information would reduce obesity. Little evidence exists suggesting that advertising is responsible for the advance in unhealthy eating.

(c) Signaling by producers (nutritional labels, health claims) and screening by consumers (reading labels accurately or using other clues to discriminate among competing food products, such as the brand name and the retailer reputation) are two possible market solutions to information problems.

---

[65] It is probably the case that in other countries—for example, the UK—the explosion in commercial TV channels has decreased the amount of time children spend watching advert-free public TV like the BBC and so they are exposed to more advertising per hour than in the past.

[66] Hastings et al. (2003).

(*d*) Transaction costs exist for information. Producing and searching for information costs money and time. These transaction costs may prevent the market from taking the solutions identified in (*c*).

Psychology and Behavioral Economics

Not all economists accept the fiction of our benchmark consumer. These skeptics are found working in the growing field of behavioral economics. Behavioral economics explores, catalogs, and rationalizes systematic deviations from the benchmark consumer. These deviations or limits on human behavior fall into three categories: bounded rationality, bounded willpower, and bounded self-interest. Bounded rationality implies that people do not have unlimited abilities to process all the information needed to make rational choices about food and health. Rather, they have inherent behavioral biases and use rules of thumb and short cuts to make decisions. Bounded willpower reflects the idea we discussed earlier that people lack self-control: we consume too much food, make rash decisions on what to eat, procrastinate on going to the gym, and so on. Bounded self-interest captures idea that people can be selfless; we are concerned about other people too. We have social preferences for emotive ideas like altruism, paternalism, and aversion to inequality.[67]

Traditionally, economic models begin with axioms about individual behavior, introduce notions of optimality within the context of a given set of preferences, and derive behavioral predictions for demand behavior that are testable at the *market* level.[68] In contrast, psychologists and behavioral economists are interested in what influences consumers' preferences and how the external environment affects preferences and behavior.[69] These two different approaches can lead to different deductions about behavior. For example, psychologists study whether people eat more when presented with larger portion sizes, and conclude that they do, based on controlled experiments.[70] They conclude that growing portion sizes have contributed to obesity. They also consider the relationship between food choices and other psychological determinants. One study[71] observed that women eat less (to behave in a more feminine way) if their male companion is desirable.

---

[67] See e.g. Mullainathan and Thaler (2000).
[68] Cutler et al. (2003).
[69] See Just et al. (2007).
[70] See e.g. Wansink (1996); Diliberti et al. (2004).
[71] Mori et al. (1987).

In contrast, economists prefer to look at the way people behave in everyday life within market-type situations. For example, when they have examined data on actual food consumption behavior (as recorded in household surveys) they have concluded that there has been no tendency for people to consume more calories per sitting. Rather, they find that extra calories are consumed by eating between meals (snacking).[72] They conclude that increased portion sizes have not contributed to obesity. The economist's assessment of the inconsistency between such findings from economists and psychologists is that the isolated decisions made outside real markets do not reflect actual behavior. And the more these food experiments are 'controlled' (in the way that clinical drug trials are), the further they are removed from the real world, in which nothing is held constant and observed behavior is the outcome of a whole range of behaviors and decisions.

Psychologists believe that economists' models of consumer behavior are overly simplistic and imply excessive rationality; economists respond by saying that this does not matter provided the models can explain real behavior in an active market exchange institution, as opposed to controlled or planned behavior, which is the focus of psychologists.[73]

Kahneman and Tversky, for instance, are psychologists who have explored the limits to the benchmark consumer.[74] They have used experimental methods to document numerous deviations from consistent choice, culminating in a descriptive behavioral model called *prospect theory*. Prospect theory allows a person to treat gains differently from equivalent losses. People value loss reductions more than they value an equivalent gain, i.e. the 50% chance of losing $1,000 has a larger utility than a 50% chance of gaining $1,000. This implies that people are risk averse when they gamble to gain wealth or health, but are risk lovers when gambling with an equivalent loss in wealth or health. In relation to obesity, this implies that people would value the prevention of a loss to status quo health more than they would value an equivalent gain in health.

Behavioral economists also focus on how consumers process information.[75] Searching for information requires effort, e.g. reading labels and looking for information over the Internet. Food purchases tend to be driven by routine rather than deliberative decisions. For these routine purchases, little or no time is spent in searching for information. Choices

---

[72] Cutler et al. (2003).

[73] For a detailed review of many findings of psychologists with respect to attitudes to food and intended food-related behavior, see Just et al. (2006).

[74] Kahneman and Tversky (1979).

[75] See East (1997, ch. 7); Solomon (2006: 308–10); Schiffman and Kanuk (2007, ch. 9).

are rather driven by habits and product recognition. Few studies exist that link consumer search and obesity. A study by Moore and Lehman (1980) shows that overweight people spent more time than others in choosing among a variety of breads with different health characteristics, although the main determinants of search behavior were price and time pressure.

We simplify our lives by relying on rules rather than basing our decisions on an accurate search and processing of all the available information. These simplifying procedures are called 'heuristics'. These rules are unconscious processes we use to save time when accessing ideas.[76] Use of heuristics is most common for frequent and low-involvement purchase decisions like food purchases. For example, a criticism of the food industry (including the fast food industry) is that their foods contain higher levels of saturated fats (which are cheaper ingredients than healthier fatty acids), sugar, and salts than similar food produced at home—or than is necessary for functional purposes. This is important when, for example, 75% of salt intake in the United Kingdom is from processed foods.[77] Given high costs of fully informing themselves about nutrition content and a tendency to make routine choices and use heuristics when buying food, an industry can 'exploit' consumers by selling foods with unhealthy ingredients that nevertheless appear healthy (e.g. 'light', 'only 10% fat', 'low-sugar').

When the industry incorporates, by accident or intention, unhealthy ingredients in food that exploit consumers' unwillingness to devote time to choosing a healthy diet, government intervention may be warranted. Policy to encourage voluntary product reformulation, for example the removal of trans fats and reduction in salt and sugar from processed foods, has been common and effective in recent years.

Just et al. (2007), for instance, discuss how the self-control problems leading to weight gain could be exacerbated by governmental policy. In the United States the government hands out food stamps monthly to participants. People with self-control problems will eat too much food during the first days rather than smoothing out consumption over the month. They could address this issue by issuing food stamps on a more regular basis, which would help people with self-control problems.

Conclusion

The key question is: what information conditions justify paternalistic government action to prevent people from eating unhealthy diets that

---

[76] Tversky and Kahneman (1974).
[77] Wanless (2004).

promote obesity? Economists argue that intervention can be warranted when information is imperfect and asymmetric. They also note that intervention is warranted when the transaction costs to process useful information are too great; or when information causes people to mis-estimate systematically the risks and benefits of eating decisions. That said, information programs aimed at reducing obesity may or may not be effective, depending on how people react to the information program. People may choose to eat better but increase risks in other areas of their lives.

Information inadequacies are a potential validation for government intervention to improve education or better inform people about the health consequences of their diets. Limited evidence, however, exists to define the empirical magnitude of the behavioral response. The existing evidence suggests minimal response to education and information. We return to these issues in discussing policy effectiveness in Chapter 4.

Obesity in Developing Countries

We set our discussion thus far in the context of a developed country consumer, noting the absence of good empirical evidence. For developing and middle-income countries, obesity is a new problem and the empirical evidence still more limited. But the methods of economics again can provide insight into the obesity question in the less developed world, especially in urban areas of middle-income countries:[78]

- rising incomes in urban areas have made overconsumption affordable;[79]

- exposure to the global mass media (linked to increasing TV ownership and viewing) and the heavy advertising of 'Western' convenience and fast foods that are more calorie-dense than traditional foods has encouraged consumption of unhealthy foods;

- more female labor force participation has increased the opportunity cost of time and increased the demand for convenience foods and eating out;

- the global economy has made vegetable oils, meat, and dairy products much cheaper than in the past;

[78] See e.g. Uusitalo et al. (2002).

[79] The growth of the middle class in developing countries has led to substantial ownership of consumer durables—televisions, but also, in a 2000 survey in Lima, Peru, of refrigerators (87% of households in the top two income deciles), cars (47%), and computers (34%). These same households consume substantially more high-value foods (Senauer and Goetz 2003).

- traditional staples are more expensive in urban areas, encouraging the switch to non-traditional diets;
- economies of scale in global food manufacturing and retailing, perhaps linked to global sourcing, have made processed food cheaper than in the past and more available;
- the increased population density associated with urbanization enables cheap eating outside the home of street foods for the poor and Western fast food for the wealthier.

Wilkinson (2004) claims that the US investments in Mexico have been concentrated in convenience and processed foods, like snacks, beverages, instant coffee, mayonnaise, and breakfast cereals. That said, it does not automatically follow that consumption of these products is higher than it would have been in the absence of foreign multinational companies.

Fast food chains such as McDonald's and Domino's and soft drink companies like Pepsi and Coke have also been blamed for unhealthy eating in developing countries and in developed countries. Pingali (2007) charts the growth of McDonald's from 951 stores in Asia and the Pacific countries in 1987 to 7,135 in 2002 and, in Latin America, from 99 to 887 over the same period. Hawkes (2005) has reviewed the marketing activities of the leading soft drink and fast food companies in developing countries, concluding that their numerous techniques to target children and teens indicate their intention of changing soft drink and fast food consumption trends over the long term. But another key factor for diets is the domestic companies that have sprung up to imitate the global brands at much lower price, and who have much higher sales.[80] Euromonitor data[81] show that soft drink sales are growing rapidly in Southeast Asian countries such as the Philippines (12% p.a.) and Indonesia (22%). The data they present shows Mexico with a per capita annual soft drink consumption of 342 liters, even higher than the US (313), UK (170), South Africa and the Philippines (about 65), China (17), and India (3).

The consequences of obesity in less developed countries could be more significant than in the developed world: people are less well educated and more open to information asymmetries about the diet–health relationship; controls on the use of unhealthy ingredients are more lax; and health systems are not equipped for dealing with health consequences of an obesity epidemic.

---

[80] Vepa (2004).
[81] Reported in Gehlhar and Regmi (2005).

Children and Families

Children are a special case in which the right of a person to choose an unhealthy lifestyle is questioned. Children are deemed unready to make a whole range of personal choices from marriage to voting and education, so it is unsurprising that governments act to influence their diets, even if direct market interventions have so far been limited.[82] Specific areas of the economist's model of food choice that cause concern when applied to children include lack of nutrition understanding, susceptibility to marketing messages, inability to foresee the near or distant future (implying more decisions that lead to immediate gratification), and an inability to perceive and balance risks. Intervention may be defensible both to reduce childhood overweight and obesity, and to affect the habits developed in childhood which are carried forward into adulthood.

Intra-Household Allocation Models

In economics, consumer theory assumes that people make their consumption choices with the aim of maximizing their own utility, conditional on an income constraint. But empirical data rarely refer to unique individuals; rather, data capture decisions within a household. Economists circumvent this shortcoming by assuming that households behave like individuals. This corresponds to assuming that each household has a single utility function which is maximized subject to a household budget constraint, i.e. the pooled income of all household members. This approach has been challenged by empirical counterevidence.[83] Not surprisingly, different people in the same household have different preference sets. Furthermore, decision making within the household may respond to varying 'power' balances. Empirically, studies on US data have shown an inverse relationship between income and obesity for adult women, but not necessarily for men and children.[84] Family structures and employment also impact on dietary patterns. Families headed by single parents were found to allocate a smaller proportion of their food budgets to vegetables and fruit as compared to married parents even after allowing for income differences. Families in which the mother is unemployed outside the house also show a smaller share of the food budget allocated to eating out and a larger share to fruit and vegetables.[85]

---

[82] See Cawley (2006).
[83] Alderman et al. (1995).
[84] Sobal and Stunkard (1989).
[85] Ziol-Guest et al. (2006).

The success of nutrition interventions targeted at individuals depends on the 'sharing rules' applied within the family. Policy implementation requires accurate knowledge of the factors determining intra-household allocation choices. A typical example is the failure of payments in the US aimed at improving the nutrition of pre-school children because parents distribute part of the extra food to other family members.[86] There are studies showing that male income earners are inclined to spend money for their own consumption, including alcohol, cigarettes, and even drugs,[87] whereas women play a larger role in the food consumption choices of the household, especially children's nutrition. For this reason, in the mid-1970s British policymakers decided to make child allowances payable in cash to mothers.[88] There is also evidence that children's body mass index and nutrient intakes are related to which household member is controlling income, as women spend a larger share of their budget on food and childcare.[89]

This opens the way to an alternative assumption in economics: income is not pooled and those in the household with larger income shares influence consumption of the other household members. The policy implication of this alternative household consumption model is that income subsidies need to be targeted to the right household member to be effective.

Economists have begun to deal with the complexity of household decision processes such as those that determine the allocation of nutrients (and health) to the different family members. Intra-household allocation models based on the collective utility function provide a basis for empirical analysis even with data sets in which the surveyed statistical unit is the household. Provided that an exclusive good can be identified for each of the household members, it becomes possible to elicit a sharing rule which synthesizes the decision process in terms of budget allocation to, and expenditure by, each family member. This opens the way to evaluating the individual response to changes in socio-economic determinants and the impact of targeted policy interventions. While the existing literature has focused on undernutrition and children,[90] the approach is also valid for evaluating policy interventions addressing overnutrition. The method could also be extended to consider other sensitive groups such as the

---

[86] Alderman et al. (1995).
[87] Alderman et al. (1995); Borelli and Perali (2003).
[88] Lundberg and Pollak (1993).
[89] Thomas (1990, 1994).
[90] Behrman and Deolalikar (1988).

elderly. We expect this to be a fruitful area for future economic research with direct relevance to policymaking.

Conclusion

Economists think differently about obesity than nutritionists. Economists stress that people are free to adapt and react to changes in relative prices set either by the marketplace or by government fiat. People do not take the world as given, which means that well-intentioned policy can be misguided. Such policies produce fewer gains at greater costs. Our review of the economic mindset has revealed four broad principles to help guide public health policies to achieve more public health at fewer costs:

Markets matter. Everyday decisions on production and consumption are subject to market forces and the interaction between demand and supply. Under the assumptions of absence of externalities, perfect information, and no excess market power, markets provide socially desirable outcomes. A comprehensive model of the consumer decision-making process shows that, given perfect information and the absence of market power, over-consumption of food resulting in obesity does not mean the market has failed.

Markets can fail. Markets fail in the presence of externalities, market power, or imperfect information. It is important to monitor whether markets fail and, if so, the likely consequences.

Relative prices matter. Regardless of whether obesity is a market failure, the household production model generates hypotheses that, if supported by evidence, can shed light on the emergence of the obesity epidemic and make predictions about future change. First, relative prices are important predictors of consumption; falling real food prices over the past twenty years and falling price of processed and fast foods relative to unprocessed foods are drivers of increased calorie intake. Second, relative time costs of goods can affect their consumption and, in the case of food, technological advances permitting mass production of processed foods and meals away from home combined with less total time available to households have been a key factor in driving consumption of processed foods, snack foods, and meals outside the home. Third, people substitute risks; advances in medical technology and reduced prevalence of smoking may have encouraged people to risk being more overweight.

83

Information campaigns are not a panacea. While consumers may rationally decide to face risky behaviors if these provide them with 'utility', a key condition for the market to work is that they are informed. Information, education, and knowledge do improve markets, but again, interventions need to anticipate the reaction of markets, because more information does not necessarily result in healthier behavior. It is unclear and, perhaps, unlikely that better information would reduce obesity. There is little evidence that advertising is responsible for the advance in unhealthy eating. Signaling by producers (nutritional labels, health claims) and screening by consumers (reading labels or using other clues to discriminate among competing food products, such as the brand name and the retailer reputation) are two possible market solutions to information problems. Transaction costs exist for information. Producing and searching for information costs money and time. These transaction costs may prevent the market agents from taking the signaling and screening actions which would solve the information problems.

References

Adelaja, A. O., R. M. Nayga, and T. C. Lauderbach (1997), 'Income and Racial Differentials in Selected Nutrient Intakes', *American Journal of Agricultural Economics*, 79/5: 1452–60.

Akerlof, G. A. (1970), 'The Market for Lemons: Quality Uncertainty and Market Mechanism', *Quarterly Journal of Economics*, 84/3: 488–500.

Alderman, H., P. A. Chiappori, L. Haddad, J. Hoddinott, and R. Kanbur (1995), 'Unitary versus Collective Models of the Household: Is it Time to Shift the Burden of Proof?', *World Bank Research Observer*, 10/1: 1–19.

Alston, J. M., J. A. Chalfant, and N. E. Piggott (2000), 'The Incidence of the Costs and Benefits of Generic Advertising', *American Journal of Agricultural Economics*, 82/3: 665–71.

—— J. W. Freebairn, and J. S. James (2001), 'Beggar-Thy-Neighbor Advertising: Theory and Application to Generic Commodity Promotion Programs', *American Journal of Agricultural Economics*, 83/4: 888–902.

Anderson, L. R., and J. M. Mellor (2007), *Predicting Health Behaviors with an Experimental Measure of Risk Preference*, College of William and Mary, Department of Economics Working Papers 59 (Williamsburg, Va.: College of William and Mary).

Becker, G. S. (1965), 'A Theory of the Allocation on Time', *Economic Journal*, 75/299: 493–517.

—— and K. M. Murphy (1988), 'A Theory of Rational Addiction', *Journal of Political Economy*, 96/4: 675–700.

Behrman, J. R., and A. B. Deolalikar (1988), 'Health and Nutrition', in C. Hollis and T. N. Srinivasan (eds), *Handbook of Development Economics* (Amsterdam: Elsevier).

—— and B. L. Wolfe (1989), 'Does More Schooling Make Women Better Nourished and Healthier? Adult Sibling Random and Fixed Effects Estimates for Nicaragua', *Journal of Human Resources*, 24/4: 644–63.

Boetel, B. L., and D. J. Liu (2003), 'Evaluating the Effect of Generic Advertising and Food Health Information within a Meat Demand System', *Agribusiness*, 19/3: 345–54.

Borelli, S., and F. Perali (2003), *Drug Consumption and Intra-Household Distribution of Resources: The Case of Qat in an African Society*, Child Working Papers 06/2003 (Turin: Center for Household, Income, Labor and Demographic Economics).

Borghans, L., and B. H. H. Golsteyn (2006), 'Time Discounting and the Body Mass Index: Evidence from the Netherlands', *Economics and Human Biology*, 4/1: 39–61.

Bretteville-Jensen, A. L. (1999), 'Addiction and Discounting', *Journal of Health Economics*, 18/4: 393–407.

Burns, C. M., R. Richman, and I. D. Caterson (1987), 'Nutrition Knowledge in the Obese and Overweight', *International Journal of Obesity*, 11/5: 485–92.

Calfee, J. E., and J. K. Pappalardo (1991), 'Public-Policy Issues in Health Claims for Foods', *Journal of Public Policy and Marketing*, 10/1: 33–53.

Cawley, J. (2006), 'Markets and Childhood Obesity Policy', *Future of Children*, 16/1: 69–88.

Chang, V. W., and D. S. Lauderdale (2005), 'Income Disparities in Body Mass Index and Obesity in the United States, 1971–2002', *Archives of Internal Medicine*, 165/18: 2122–8.

Chen, S. N., J. F. Shogren, P. F. Orazem, and T. D. Crocker (2002), 'Prices and Health: Identifying the Effects of Nutrition, Exercise, and Medication Choices on Blood Pressure', *American Journal of Agricultural Economics*, 84/4: 990–1002.

Chesher, A. (1997), 'Diet Revealed? Semiparametric Estimation of Nutrient Intake Age Relationships', *Journal of the Royal Statistical Society*, ser. A: *Statistics in Society*, 160: 389–420.

Chou, S. Y., M. Grossman, and H. Saffer (2002), *An Economic Analysis of Adult Obesity: Results from the Behavioral Risk Factor Surveillance System*, NBER Working Papers 9247 (Cambridge, Mass.: National Bureau of Economic Research).

—— —— —— (2004), 'An Economic Analysis of Adult Obesity: Results from the Behavioral Risk Factor Surveillance System', *Journal of Health Economics*, 23/3: 565–87.

Chung, C. J., and S. L. Myers (1999), 'Do the Poor Pay More for Food? An Analysis of Grocery Store Availability and Food Price Disparities', *Journal of Consumer Affairs*, 33/2: 276–96.

Cutler, D. M., E. L. Glaeser, and J. M. Shapiro (2003), 'Why Have Americans Become More Obese?', *Journal of Economic Perspectives*, 17/3: 93–118.

de Laat, J., and A. S. Sanz (2006), *Working Women, Men's Home Time and Lowest-Low Fertility*, ISER Working Paper 2006–23.

Diliberti, N., P. L. Bordi, M. T. Conklin, L. S. Roe, and B. J. Rolls (2004), 'Increased Portion Size Leads to Increased Energy Intake in a Restaurant Meal', *Obesity Research*, 12/3: 562–8.

Drewnowski, A., and S. E. Specter (2004), 'Poverty and Obesity: The Role of Energy Density and Energy Costs', *American Journal of Clinical Nutrition*, 79/1: 6–16.

Duecy, E. (2006), 'Chain QSR Market Share Growing in Big European Markets', *Nation's Restaurant News*, 40/37: 16.

East, R. (1997), *Consumer Behavior: Advances and Applications in Marketing* (New York: Prentice Hall).

Ervin, R. B., J. D. Wright, C. Y. Wang, and J. Kennedy-Stephenson (2004), 'Dietary Intake of Fats and Fatty Acids for the United States Population: 1999–2000', *Advance Data from Vital and Health Statistics* 348 (Hyattsville, Mass.: National Center for Health Statistics).

Estrin, S., and D. E. W. Laidler (1995), *Introduction to Microeconomics* (New York: Prentice Hall).

Field, A. E., S. B. Austin, M. W. Gillman, B. Rosner, H. R. Rockett, and G. A. Colditz (2004), 'Snack Food Intake Does Not Predict Weight Change among Children and Adolescents', *International Journal of Obesity and Related Metabolic Disorders*, 28/10: 1210–16.

Filozof, C., M. C. Fernandez Pinilla, and A. Fernandez-Cruz (2004), 'Smoking Cessation and Weight Gain', *Obesity Reviews*, 5/2: 95–103.

Flegal, K. M., R. P. Troiano, E. R. Pamuk, R. J. Kuczmarski, and S. M. Campbell (1995), 'The Influence of Smoking Cessation on the Prevalence of Overweight in the United States', *New England Journal of Medicine*, 333/18: 1165–70.

Frederick, S., G. Loewenstein, and T. O'Donoghue (2002), 'Time Discounting and Time Preference: A Critical Review', *Journal of Economic Literature*, 40/2: 351–401.

Fuchs, V. R. (1982), 'Time Preference and Health: An Exploratory Study', in Fuchs (ed.), *Economic Aspects of Health* (Chicago: University of Chicago Press).

Gardner, B. (2003), 'US Food Quality Standards: Fix for Market Failure or Costly Anachronism?', *American Journal of Agricultural Economics*, 85/3: 725–30.

Garretson, J. A., and S. Burton (2000), 'Effects of Nutrition Facts Panel Values, Nutrition Claims, and Health Claims on Consumer Attitudes, Perceptions of Disease-Related Risks, and Trust', *Journal of Public Policy and Marketing*, 19/2: 213–27.

Gehlhar, M., and A. Regmi (2005), *Factors Shaping Global Food Markets*, Agricultural Information Bulletin 794 (Washington: ERS-USDA).

Greenland, P. (2001), 'Beating High Blood Pressure with Low-Sodium DASH', *New England Journal of Medicine*, 344/1: 53–5.

Gruber, J., and M. Frakes (2006), 'Does Falling Smoking Lead to Rising Obesity?', *Journal of Health Economics*, 25/2: 183–97.

Hankey, C., A. Lee, W. Leslie, M. Lean, and L. McCombie (2004), 'Nutrition Knowledge in the Overweight and Obese Does Not Predict Inclination to Attempt Weight Loss', *International Journal of Obesity*, 28: S136.

Harrison, G. W., M. I. Lau, and M. B. Williams (2002), 'Estimating Individual Discount Rates in Denmark: A Field Experiment', *American Economic Review*, 92/5: 1606–17.

Hastings, G., M. Stead, L. McDermott, A. Forsyth, A. M. MacKintosh, M. Rayner, C. Godfrey, M. Caraher, and K. Angus (2003), *Review of Research on the Effects of Food Promotion to Children*, Report prepared for the Food Standards Agency (Strathclyde: University of Strathclyde, Centre for Social Marketing).

Hawkes, C. (2005), 'The Role of Foreign Direct Investment in the Nutrition Transition', *Public Health Nutrition*, 8/4: 357–65.

Huston, S. J., and M. S. Finke (2003), 'Diet Choice and the Role of Time Preference', *Journal of Consumer Affairs*, 37/1: 143–60.

Iida, K., and R. N. Proctor (2004), 'Learning from Philip Morris: Japan Tobacco's Strategies regarding Evidence of Tobacco Health Harms as Revealed in Internal Documents from the American Tobacco Industry', *The Lancet*, 363/9423: 1820–4.

Jargon, J. (2006), 'The King is Lurking', *Crain's Chicago Business*, 29/39: 3–10.

Just, D. R., L. Mancino, and B. Wansink (2007), *Could Behavioral Economics Help Improve Diet Quality for Nutrition Assistance Program Participants?*, Economic Research Report 43 (Washington: US Department of Agriculture, Economic Research Service).

Kahneman, D., and A. Tversky (1979), 'Prospect Theory: An Analysis of Decision under Risk', *Econometrica*, 47/2: 263–91.

Kan, K., and W. D. Tsai (2004), 'Obesity and Risk Knowledge', *Journal of Health Economics*, 23/5: 907–34.

Kenkel, D. S. (1991), 'Health Behavior, Health Knowledge, and Schooling', *Journal of Political Economy*, 99/2: 287–305.

Komlos, J., P. K. Smith, and B. Bogin (2004), 'Obesity and the Rate of Time Preference: Is there a Connection?', *Journal of Biosocial Science*, 36/2: 209–19.

Kuchler, F., E. Golan, J. N. Variyam, and S. R. Crutchfield (2005), 'Obesity Policy and the Law of Unintended Consequences', *Amber Waves*, 3/3: 26–33.

Lakdawalla, D., and T. J. Philipson (2002), *The Growth of Obesity and Technological Change: A Theoretical and Empirical Examination*, NBER Working Papers 8946 (Cambridge, Mass.: National Bureau of Economic Research).

Lang, T., and M. Heasman (2004), *Food Wars* (London: Earthscan).

Lenfant, C. (1996), 'High Blood Pressure: Some Answers, New Questions, Continuing Challenges', *Journal of the American Medical Association*, 275/20: 1604–6.

Levy, A. (2002), 'Rational Eating: Can it Lead to Overweightness or Underweightness?', *Journal of Health Economics*, 21/5: 887–99.

Levy, A. S., and R. C. Stokes (1987), 'Effects of a Health Promotion Advertising Campaign on Sales of Ready-to-Eat Cereals', *Public Health Reports*, 102/4: 398–403.

Louriero, M. L. and R. M. Nayga (2005), 'International Dimensions of Obesity and Overweight Related Problems: An Economics Perspective', *American Journal of Agricultural Economics*, 87/5: 1147–53.

Lundberg, S., and R. A. Pollak (1993), 'Separate Spheres Bargaining and the Marriage Market', *Journal of Political Economy*, 101/6: 988–1010.

McCormick, B., and I. Stone (2007), 'Economic Costs of Obesity and the Case for Government Intervention', *Obesity Reviews*, 8: 161–4.

Mazzocchi, M., and W. B. Traill (2007), 'Calories, Obesity and Health in OECD Countries', Paper presented at the 81st Annual Conference of the Agricultural Economics Society, University of Reading, 2–4 Apr.

Midgley, J. P., A. G. Matthew, C. M. T. Greenwood, and A. G. Logan (1996), 'Effect of Reduced Dietary Sodium on Blood Pressure: A Meta-Analysis of Randomized Controlled Trials', *JAMA: Journal of the American Medical Association*, 275/20: 1590–7.

Molarius, A. (2003), 'The Contribution of Lifestyle Factors to Socioeconomic Differences in Obesity in Men and Women: A Population-Based Study in Sweden', *European Journal of Epidemiology*, 18/3: 227–34.

—— J. C. Seidell, S. Sans, J. Tuomilehto, and K. Kuulasmaa (2000), 'Educational Level, Relative Body Weight, and Changes in their Association over 10 Years: An International Perspective from the WHO MONICA Project', *American Journal of Public Health*, 90/8: 1260–8.

Moore, W. L., and D. R. Lehmann (1980), 'Individual Differences in Search Behavior for a Nondurable', *Journal of Consumer Research*, 7/3: 296–307.

Mori, D., P. Pliner, and S. Chaiken (1987), 'Eating Lightly and the Self-Presentation of Femininity', *Journal of Personality and Social Psychology*, 53/4: 693–702.

Mullainathan, S., and R. Thaler (2000), *Behavioral Economics*, NBER Working Papers 7948 (Cambridge, Mass.: National Bureau of Economic Research).

Nayga, R. M. (2000), 'Schooling, Health Knowledge and Obesity', *Applied Economics*, 32/7: 815–22.

Oliver, J. E., and T. Lee (2005), 'Public Opinion and the Politics of Obesity in America', *Journal of Health Politics Policy and Law*, 30/5: 923–54.

Philipson, T. J. (2001), 'The World-Wide Growth in Obesity: An Economic Research Agenda', *Health Economics*, 10/1: 1–7.

—— and R. A. Posner (1999), 'The Long-Run Growth in Obesity as a Function of Technological Change', *Perspectives in Biology and Medicine*, 46/3: S87–S107.

Pickett, K. E., S. Kelly, E. Brunner, T. Lobstein, and R. G. Wilkinson (2005), 'Wider Income Gaps, Wider Waistbands? An Ecological Study of Obesity and Income Inequality', *Journal of Epidemiology and Community Health*, 59/8: 670–4.

Picone, G., and F. Sloan (2003), 'Smoking Cessation and Lifestyle Changes', *Forum for Health Economics and Policy*, 6 (Berkeley Electronic Press).

Pingali, P. (2007), 'Westernization of Asian Diets and the Transformation of Food Systems: Implications for Research and Policy', *Food Policy*, 32/3: 281–98.

Pitt, M. M., and M. R. Rosenzweig (1986), 'Agricultural Prices, Food Consumption and the Health and Productivity of Farmers', in I. Singh, L. Squire, and J. Strauss (eds), *Agricultural Household Models: Extensions, Applications, and Policy* (Baltimore: Johns Hopkins University Press).

Reardon, T., and J. A. Berdegue (2002), 'The Rapid Rise of Supermarkets in Latin America: Challenges and Opportunities for Development', *Development Policy Review*, 20/4: 371–88.

—— C. P. Timmer, C. B. Barrett, and J. Berdegue (2003), 'The Rise of Supermarkets in Africa, Asia, and Latin America', *American Journal of Agricultural Economics*, 85/5: 1140–6.

Regmi, A., M. S. Deepak, J. L. Seale, Jr, and J. Bernstein (2001), *Cross-Country Analysis of Food Consumption Patterns*, WRS 01-01 (Washington: USDA-ERS).

Richards, T. J., and P. M. Patterson (2006), 'Native American Obesity: An Economic Model of the "Thrifty Gene" Theory', *American Journal of Agricultural Economics*, 88/3: 542–60.

Rodu, B., B. Stegmayr, S. Nasic, P. Cole, and K. Asplund (2004), 'The Influence of Smoking and Smokeless Tobacco Use on Weight amongst Men', *Journal of Internal Medicine*, 255/1: 102–7.

Schiffman, L. G., and L. L. Kanuk (2007), *Consumer Behavior* (Upper Saddle River, NJ: Prentice Hall).

Seiders, K., and R. D. Petty (2004), 'Obesity and the Role of Food Marketing: A Policy Analysis of Issues and Remedies', *Journal of Public Policy and Marketing*, 23/2: 153–69.

Senauer, B., and L. Goetz (2003), *The Growing Middle Class in Developing Countries and the Market for High-Value Food Products*, Working Paper 03-02 (Minneapolis: University of Minnesota, Food Industry Center).

Shogren, J. F. (2005), 'Economics of Diet and Health: Research Challenges', *Food Economics: Acta Agriculturae Scandinavica*, sect. C, 2/3: 117–27.

—— and T. D. Crocker (1999), 'Risk and its Consequences', *Journal of Environmental Economics and Management*, 37/1: 44–51.

Silberberg, E. (1985), 'Nutrition and the Demand for Tastes', *Journal of Political Economy*, 93/5: 881–900.

Skinner, T., H. Miller, and C. Bryant (2005), 'The Literature on the Economic Causes of and Policy Responses to Obesity', *Food Economics: Acta Agriculturae Scandinavica*, sect. C, 2/3: 128–37.

Smith, P. K., B. Bogin, and D. Bishai (2005), 'Are Time Preference and Body Mass Index Associated? Evidence from the National Longitudinal Survey of Youth', *Economics and Human Biology*, 3/2: 259–70.

Sobal, J., and A. J. Stunkard (1989), 'Socioeconomic Status and Obesity: A Review of the Literature', *Psychological Bulletin*, 105/2: 260–75.

Solomon, M. R. (2006), *Consumer Behavior: Buying, Having and Being* (Upper Saddle River, NJ: Prentice Hall).

Story, M., and S. French (2004), 'Food Advertising and Marketing Directed at Children and Adolescents in the US', *International Journal of Behavioral Nutrition and Physical Activity*, 1/1: 3–17.

Strauss, J. (1986), 'Does Better Nutrition Raise Farm Productivity', *Journal of Political Economy*, 94/2: 297–320.

Subramanian, S., and A. Deaton (1996), 'The Demand for Food and Calories', *Journal of Political Economy*, 104/1: 133–62.

Swan, G. (2004), 'Findings from the Latest National Diet and Nutrition Survey', *Proceedings of the Nutrition Society*, 63/4: 505–12.

Teisl, M. F., N. E. Bockstael, and A. Levy (2001), 'Measuring the Welfare Effects of Nutrition Information', *American Journal of Agricultural Economics*, 83/1: 133–49.

Theil, H., Ching-Fan Chung, and J. L. Seale, Jr (1989), *International Evidence on Consumption Patterns* (Greenwich, Conn.: JAI Press).

Thomas, D. (1990), 'Intrahousehold Resource-Allocation: An Inferential Approach', *Journal of Human Resources*, 25/4: 635–64.

—— (1994), 'Like Father, Like Son—Like Mother, Like Daughter: Parental Resources and Child Height', *Journal of Human Resources*, 29/4: 950–88.

Thomson Datastream (2007), <http://www.datastream.com>.

Traill, W. B. (2006), 'The Rapid Rise of Supermarkets?', *Development Policy Review*, 24/2: 163–74.

Tversky, A., and D. Kahneman (1974), 'Judgment under Uncertainty: Heuristics and Biases', *Science*, 185/4157: 1124–31.

Uusitalo, U., P. Pietinen, and P. Puska (2002), 'Dietary Transition in Developing Countries: Challenges for Chronic Disease Prevention', in D. Yach and P. Puska (eds), *Globalization, Diets and Non-Communicable Diseases* (Geneva: World Health Organization).

Variyam, J. N., J. Blaylock, B. H. Lin, K. Ralston, and D. Smallwood (1999), 'Mother's Nutrition Knowledge and Children's Dietary Intakes', *American Journal of Agricultural Economics*, 81/2: 373–84.

Vepa, S. S. (2004), 'Impact of Globalization on the Food Consumption of Urban India', *FAO Food and Nutrition Paper*, 83: 215–30.

Verbeke, W. (2005), 'Agriculture and the Food Industry in the Information Age', *European Review of Agricultural Economics*, 32/3: 347–68.

Vuchinich, R. E., and C. A. Simpson (1999), 'Delayed Reward Discounting in Alcohol Abuse', in F. J. Chaloupka, M. Grossman, W. K. Bickel, and H. Saffer (eds), *The Economic Analysis of Substance Use and Abuse: An Integration of Econometric and Behavioral Economic Research* (Chicago: University of Chicago Press).

Wanless, D. (2004), *Securing Good Health for the Whole Population: Final Report* (Norwich: HMSO).

Wansink, B. (1996), 'Can Package Size Accelerate Usage Volume?', *Journal of Marketing*, 60/3: 1–14.

Weber, E. U., A. R. Blais, and N. E. Betz (2002), 'A Domain-Specific Risk-Attitude Scale: Measuring Risk Perceptions and Risk Behaviors', *Journal of Behavioral Decision Making*, 15/4: 263–90.

Wilkinson, J. (2004), 'The Food Processing Industry, Globalization and Developing Countries', *Electronic Journal of Agricultural and Development Economics*, 1/2: 184–201.

Yach, D., D. Stuckler, and K. D. Brownell (2006), 'Epidemiologic and Economic Consequences of the Global Epidemics of Obesity and Diabetes', *Nature Medicine*, 12/1: 62–6.

Zhang, L. E. I., and I. Rashad (2008), 'Obesity and Time Preference: The Health Consequences of Discounting the Future', *Journal of Biosocial Science*, 40/1: 97–113.

Ziol-Guest, K. M., T. DeLeire, and A. Kalil (2006), 'The Allocation of Food Expenditure in Married- and Single-Parent Families', *Journal of Consumer Affairs*, 40/2: 347–71.

Zywicki, T. J., D. Holt, and M. K. Ohlhausen (2004), 'Obesity and Advertising Policy', *George Mason Law Review*, 12/4: 979–1011.

3

Economic Evaluation Tools for Evidence-Based Policymaking

Imagine a situation in which everyone is well educated, well informed, and self-controlled, and the costs of obesity are borne only by obese people. People either pay their own medical expenses or pay health insurance whose costs reflect their risks. This implies that society does not bear any 'external' medical costs. Similarly, less job productivity due to obesity implies lower wages (see Box 3.1 for a discussion of this issue). Assume that all markets operate under perfect competition so that the prices of all goods accurately reflect the cost of the resources used to produce them. Now suppose that a government agency decides to 'induce' people to eat less chocolate and more fruit and vegetables so that we all lose weight and become healthier.

The economist would ask whether this inducement would be justified by considering its ratio of costs-to-benefits. From an economic perspective, the answer is 'no': the cost–benefit ratio is not just small, it would be negative. While it costs money to implement this new regulation, no benefits are produced. Rather the benefits are negative. But how can benefits be negative even though there are fewer overweight people, better health, and reduced medical expenditures? The reason is that people were doing exactly what they wanted (i.e. maximizing their own utility) before the intervention. By definition, they must now be less satisfied by being *induced* to change their behavior to purchase a less preferred set of goods. The loss in utility from being unable to select one's favorite bundle of food items exceeds the gain in utility from being healthier; otherwise, they would have made the opposite decision before the intervention.

But policymakers frequently assume that all gains in lifespan and health status are gains to society. They do not address the point that people may have previously chosen the probability of a shorter life or less health rather

---

Box 3.1. Additional costs borne by obese people

Data suggest that obese white females in America earn 17% less than their normal-weight counterparts.[1] On average, a larger body mass index (BMI) is associated with lower salaries for both males and females,[2] but obese males seem to fill the wage gap by turning to jobs in which size may be an advantage or accept better-paid but riskier jobs. Furthermore, the wage offset for obese women occurs because of higher insurance premiums paid by the employer; but this wage offset exceeds the incremental health care costs of obese females, but not for males.[3] For Europe difference also emerges between male and female workers.[4] Again, penalization in employment and wages seems to be associated with the level of employer-provided health care, suggesting that the employee is being made to pay the cost he or she imposes on the company. A study for France[5] also shows that obese people have a hard time finding a job. Discrimination could be greater in countries in which obesity rates are lower, as a consequence of stronger societal stigmatization.

These findings raise a controversial issue. Economic theory suggests that higher costs and lower wages for obese people should provide incentive for them to lose weight. In contrast, the financial discrimination of overweight people raises political and ethical concerns, especially in countries like the US, in which they are the majority of the population. To illustrate the political paradox, Carpenter (2006) shows how the Americans with Disabilities Act and a 1993 court ruling have increased employment for obese men and women relative to non-obese people.

---

than giving up utility by eating more cheaply or more pleasurably. People cannot have it both ways. So, if overweight and obesity arise from free will, why should governments intervene to fight it? Why is obesity so prominent in governments' policy agendas?

Recall from Chapter 2 that markets can fail to provide a socially optimal outcome if there is a distortion between private and social welfare. Social welfare is greatest when each person bears all of the costs of their choices without imposing unwanted costs on the rest of the society. Negative externalities and market failure arise when obesity generates costs for non-obese people. Chapter 2 discussed how markets fail to price all the costs because many medical costs and employment expenses are borne by society, not just those who are obese. If people do not consider all the costs of their decisions, government intervention in markets may work to improve social welfare—provided the social benefits of intervention exceed social costs.

---

[1] See references in Finkelstein et al. (2005) and Cawley (2004).

[2] Baum and Ford (2004); Pagán and Dávila (1997).

[3] Bhattacharya and Bundorf (2005). Instead, Wada and Tekin (2007) argue that using a fat composition index rather than the BMI leads to consistent results and both males and females experience wage reductions.

[4] Garcia and Quintana-Domeque (2007).

[5] Paraponaris et al. (2005).

We now distinguish more carefully between the social and private costs of obesity. The social costs are those caused by the externality that people impose on others when they are overweight; the private costs are those they bear themselves through lower wages, ill health, and premature death. We discuss the likely magnitude of the social costs, and the costs and benefits which should be counted when evaluating policy interventions.

We begin the chapter with a review of the various efforts to quantify the social costs in order to have a view of their social importance. We proceed to review methods employed by public health professionals and economists to compute the benefits of intervention, essentially through the development of measures of the utility associated with states of ill health and premature death. These can be used in ex ante policy evaluation (decision rules before a policy is implemented to determine whether it would be good value for money) and in ex post evaluation (determining afterwards whether a policy was cost-effective), and we discuss modern economic tools for such evaluation.

Measures of the Direct and Indirect Costs to Society of Obesity

Quantifying costs also allows one to predict the benefits of obesity reduction policies. Bad nutrition and lifestyle choices generate obesity, obesity leads to bad health, and bad health generates costs to individuals and society. If one accepts this model,[6] the costs of obesity to society can be assessed through a quantification of its direct costs (to the health care system) and indirect costs (defined as lost productivity).

In this model the main obstacle to monetizing outcomes is the incomplete evidence about the actual link between obesity and obesity-related disease. For example, we know that the prevalence of diabetes is increasing.[7] It is not straightforward, however, to determine why: is it the relative contribution of obesity, bad nutrition, and other lifestyle factors, or simply increased life expectancy? Similarly, different lifestyle factors provoke heart conditions, including smoking and lack of exercise, and it proves difficult to separate them from the obesity component. It is common in the public health literature to measure the medical cost of obesity by attributing to it a share of relevant non-communicable diseases; for example, hypothetically, half

---

[6] For example, Oliver (2006) argues bad nutrition choices generate bad health, but obesity is not necessarily the missing link.

[7] See Wild et al. (2004); Roglic et al. (2005).

of type II diabetes cases are caused by obesity. The assessment of indirect costs, like reduced productivity, may be also based on comparison of the number of days of work missed through ill health by obese and normal-weight people, assuming they are the same in all other respects.

A detailed study by the National Audit Office (2001) in England gives an estimate of the medical costs of overweight and obesity of about £500 million ($1 billion). This report has detailed estimates of the cost share attributable to food for the various diseases. For example, 36% of hyper-tension cases are estimated to be attributable to obesity, 47% of type II diabetes cases, and 29% of colon cancer cases. After allowing for the cost per case and the total number of cases, the hypertension-related share of the total cost of obesity is 29%, diabetes 26%, and colon cancer 2%. Around 50% of these costs are for prescriptions, 40% are hospital costs, and 10% are GP (doctor) costs.

The recent government Foresight Report[8] designed to think about the long-term consequences of obesity accepts £1 billion (about $2 billion) as the best estimate of the current medical costs of overweight and obesity in England and, using a model to project obesity forwards to 2050, estimates that the health care cost would rise to £7.1 billion if current trends con-tinued, representing a rise in the share of health care costs attributable to overweight and obesity from 1.4% to 10.1%. £1 billion represents about 0.1% of national income (GDP).

Popkin et al. (2006) allow dietary factors to have direct impacts on health, as well as the indirect effects caused by obesity. For example, eating more fruit and vegetables and whole grains affects health directly by reducing cancer and indirectly by reducing obesity. High intake of satur-ated and trans fats can have negative direct health effects. For China, Popkin and his colleagues estimate that the combined direct and indirect effects of diet contribute $3.9 billion to medical costs. A further $2.2 billion are imposed by low levels of physical activity, of which about a third are through the obesity pathway. In total, diet-related costs represent about 0.3% of GDP.

The impact that weight *loss* has on medical costs remains uncertain. But this information is needed to calculate the cost–benefit ratio of policy interventions to change diet and reduce weight. Without this informa-tion, one must assume that a person who reduces his weight, say from BMI 30 to 25, has the same medical costs as someone whose BMI has always been 25, an uncomfortable assumption. Wolf (2002) reviews research

---

[8] McPherson et al. (2007).

which suggests that the cost of weight-reducing pharmaceuticals may be offset by savings in drugs to treat hypertension, diabetes, and hyperlipidemia, which decrease owing to weight loss. But more evidence is needed; it is unlikely that the weight–cost relationship associated with weight gain is symmetrical with that for weight loss. Prevention may be more cost-effective than cure.

Wolf and Colditz (1998) have calculated the medical costs of obesity for the US. Their results are dated (1995 data), however, and probably underestimate the current position. They estimate that the annual medical costs of obesity (not overweight) are between 5.5% and 7% of total medical expenditure.

In estimating the costs of obesity, one should control for all other individual characteristics correlated with obesity which might wrongly be attributed solely to obesity by a simple comparison of the medical costs of obese and normal-weight individuals. These include social deprivation, smoking, and alcohol consumption. One method to control for such factors is in a multiple regression framework. Finkelstein et al. (2003) use individual medical expenditure data (from the Medical Expenditure Panel Survey) combined with self-reported height and weight (to obtain BMI), and use regression analysis on US adults to estimate medical expenditure as a function of demographic variables (race, age, region, income) and dummy variables for overweight and obesity. The regression analysis shows the extra medical costs associated with obesity and overweight while controlling for demographic factors (but not smoking and drinking). They find that the additional medical costs of the overweight are 11.4%; for the obese, the additional costs are 37.4%. Combined with overweight and obesity prevalence data this implies that 3.7% and 5.3% of total medical expenditures are associated with overweight and obesity.

Finkelstein et al. also break down the additional costs attributable to excess weight. Out-of-pocket expenditure, which includes payments by the uninsured and payment not covered by insurance, is 11.1% higher for overweight individuals and 26.1% higher for obese individuals compared to normal-weight individuals. The gap is higher if one considers costs covered by the main public insurance schemes, Medicaid and Medicare. Medicaid is a publicly funded program for low-income individuals and families who meet some further requirements, such as children, pregnant women, seniors, and people with disabilities, to cover (partially or fully) their medical expenses and health services. Medicare is also a public insurance scheme, entirely funded by the federal government, which mainly supports those over 65, who represent one quarter of the US population. Obese individuals eligible for the Medicaid insurance category face costs that are 39.1% higher than their normal-weight counterparts (36.8% for Medicare). The costs of these programs are borne by all tax-payers, including slim taxpaying workers, thus the higher spending for publicly insured individuals can be regarded as an obesity externality.[9]

Critics contend that studies which calculate the annual costs of obesity have not accounted for the impact of obesity on life expectancy. If a person's annual medical costs are twice as high per year, but he lives half as long as the average person, then his medical cost burden on society is *neutral.* This remains an unsettled issue: studies suggest that the number of years of costly disability associated with obesity is not much different from that for the non-obese population; obese people usually do not die at retirement age. For example, Allison et al. (1999) estimate that 4.3% of lifetime health care costs are associated with obesity, slightly below the 5.3% annual figure of Finkelstein et al. But a recent study in the Nether-lands suggests that because obese people die younger and with lower terminal medical costs than normal-weight people, their cumulative med-ical costs from age 20 on are $371,000 compared to $417,000 for those of normal weight.[10]

Tucker et al. (2006) developed a health cost simulation model based on US data. They account for both annual medical costs and life expectancy for black and white males and females over a wide range of BMIs from 24 to 44 and over a range of ages. Life expectancy for 60-year-old white females peaks at a BMI of about 29 and then falls steadily; but for black females and males, life expectancy continues to rise to a BMI of around 40. For white males, life expectancy falls steadily throughout the BMI range but at the age of 60 a white male with BMI 24 has a life expectancy of 21 years, only three years longer than one with a BMI of 44. Despite these surprising relationships, medical costs associated with overweight and obesity rise almost linearly throughout the BMI range, albeit not rapidly.

The UK National Audit Survey study[11] also estimated the indirect costs of obesity. They found that 6% of deaths are obesity-related, and more than a third occurred before retirement age. They computed total lost earnings, equaling £827 million (around $1.6 billion) in 1998. To this was added £1.3 billion ($2.6 billion) for days missed from work through sickness related to obesity. They recognized that this is likely to be an

---

[9] Finkelstein et al. (2003).
[10] Van Baal et al. (2008).
[11] National Audit Office (2001).

underestimate of sickness because medical certificates are not required for the first five days of illness. The figure is about 0.2% of GDP, the same as costs attributable to health care. The UK Foresight study,[12] however, argues that there is little certainty about this figure, which could be as high as £10 billion per year ($20 billion).[13]

Summary

Seven lessons emerge from our review of the costs of obesity:

1. If our interest is to focus on external costs of obesity—those imposed on others as a by-product of private consumption decisions, we should focus on medical (direct) and employment (indirect) costs. Evidence suggests that medical costs of overweight and obesity may amount to 5% of health care costs in the US, less in the UK, and presumably less still in countries with lower obesity prevalence. In terms of GDP, medical costs of overweight and obesity are less that 0.5%.

2. Estimates of the medical costs of obesity depend on the prevalence of obesity and the sophistication of a country's medical system. A country with a primitive health care system that does not treat the disease (or its manifestations like cardiovascular disease or diabetes) will have low medical costs associated with obesity but may find itself with high indirect costs as people take more days off work through illness. To our knowledge no one has measured the trade-offs between direct and indirect costs.

3. The medical costs of obesity have generally been measured within an epidemiological framework. This approach attributes a share of the prevalence of each disease to diet and apportions to diet that share of the costs of treating the disease. But the method assumes that the various causes of a disease are independent, which is unlikely. For example, an obese smoker's risks from coronary heart disease might not equal the sum of the risks to an obese non-smoker and a normal-weight smoker. Significant interactions exist. Given that risk factors are clustered in disadvantaged social

---

[12] McPherson et al. (2007).

[13] Economists still debate about whether these are genuine costs to society. If an employee is sick, does the productivity of the firm suffer proportionately or do other employees work longer and harder to compensate? And if a person dies before retirement, are his or her lost earnings wholly a cost to society or is the cost to society limited to the share he or she would have paid as taxes? And should this amount in any case be offset by any savings in state pension payments?

groups, these interactions could be economically important. Thus, a statistical approach which is able to single out the specific effect of obesity after accounting for all other risk factors is preferred. While the limited statistical evidence available today suggests that the epidemiological and statistical methods produce similar results, disentangling these synergic impacts remains a high research priority.

4. Popkin recognizes that one should account for direct impacts of dietary components (diet quality) on health as well as indirect impacts through obesity. Direct impacts can be substantial.

5. Measuring lifetime medical costs rather than annual medical costs is appropriate. Limited research is equivocal as to whether lifetime costs of obese people exceed those for normal-weight people, so this is an important area for future research. Much of the policy debate surrounding obesity relates to health care costs, so knowing whether they are positively or negatively associated with obesity is vital to evidence-based policymaking.

6. Data on how medical costs change as BMI increases are scarce. Normally the traditional cut-off for obesity is BMI >30. This is because the normal approach to measuring medical costs is based on the epidemiological approach and there does not exist a dose–response relationship between BMI and disease prevalence. In theory, finer gradations are possible using the regression approach; in practice, this still needs to be explored. Given that life expectancy is little affected by BMI below 30, more work on relationships between BMI and medical treatment for BMI between 30 and 40 is needed. More research is also needed to understand the symmetry in the relationship between medical costs and changing BMI.

7. Researchers disagree on the appropriateness of considering indirect costs to the economy resulting from lost productivity caused by days off sick and early death. It is unclear if a person who is off work for a few days causes their employer's productivity to suffer proportionately. Nor is it obvious that a premature death represents a drop in income per head for the surviving population. One could argue that a country's earlier investment in a person's education and training would not have been fully repaid if they died early. The quoted figures for indirect costs, such as from the UK National Audit Office or Popkin's study in China, put the indirect costs above the direct medical costs, so this is an important conceptual and empirical issue.

Evidence-Based Interventions and their Costs and Benefits

We just examined the probable magnitude of the direct medical costs and indirect costs to the economy of overweight and obesity. These costs are substantial but do they justify public intervention to change public behavior to reduce obesity? From the economic perspective, this depends whether the benefits of the intervention outweigh the costs.

The costs of intervention are measured as the sum of compliance and other costs to firms (e.g. costs of reformulation, labeling, lost advertising revenue, and lost demand) and costs to government of regulation (bureaucratic and costs of inspection and other monitoring). Governments sometimes go further than this and require specific assessments of the impact of interventions on small firms, sustainability, regional employment, and gender equality, though these are rarely quantified.

Measuring the benefits of intervention is conceptually more complex. At its simplest, benefits are measured as medical costs and productivity losses avoided due to the intervention, but even this requires an assessment of the impact of the intervention on diets (in the short and long terms), the impact of diets on obesity (and over what time period), and the impact of obesity on health (again taking into account the lag between obesity and health outcomes). Future outcomes should then be discounted, as we discussed in Chapter 2.

Economists believe that the benefits of intervention should be broadened to recognize and measure the utility people forgo when they are ill or die prematurely. But utility is not easily quantified and, even if it could be, how does one compare a unit of utility (a *util*) with a monetary cost? Two possible solutions are to find out how much people are *willing to pay*, and to sidestep the issue by ensuring that the same amount of money is spent in providing one util of utility by all interventions.

We remind readers to question whether an intervention to reduce obesity really increases utility. If someone is overweight as a result of taking a utility-maximizing decision based on health risks, intervention reduces utility by definition. Regulation forces people to move away from their preferred bundle of consumption goods, health, and leisure to a less preferred package so that even if people are *healthier*, they are not necessarily *happier*. There are instances when this is a reasonable argument, others when it is not. It depends whether people are overweight because they are poorly informed or poorly educated, or because they have made unhealthy choices even though they were informed and educated. One might argue, for example, that nutrition education and labeling (together permitting informed choice) are examples of interventions taken to correct informational market failures. If as a consequence people are enabled and respond by choosing a healthier diet, their utility increases. The usual complex measurement questions to be addressed are: how much do people adjust their behavior, how does this affect their health, how much utility does this give them, and is this enough to warrant the extra costs imposed on industry and government? The same argument can be made about funding research to develop, say, trans fat free canola oil. People are provided with an extra choice; if they choose it, they do so because they expect increased utility. Is the extra utility, associated with the health benefits, sufficient to outweigh the costs of the research? In contrast, fat taxes and thin subsidies are intended solely to change behavior and are much harder to justify as enhancing utility, though they may still be justified in terms of correcting an externality—the medical and productivity costs imposed on society.

We see the importance of distinguishing between private and social benefits in the analysis of policy interventions: benefits can accrue either to everyone in society or to just a few. Clarity is crucial in distinguishing what is appropriate to measure and under what circumstances.

In relation to private benefits, economists' preferred measures are (i) how much people would be willing to pay for adopting the intervention, or (ii) the amount of money people would be willing to accept in compensation if the intervention is not adopted. These measures are called the *willingness-to-pay* (WTP) and *willingness-to-accept* (WTA). In theory, these measures of value are similar for goods with close substitutes (bread, milk), but can differ significantly when the good has few substitutes (e.g. your health).

A person's WTP is the maximum he or she would pay for policy change, which would leave them indifferent as to whether the intervention took place. If they actually had to pay more, they would be worse off (in utility terms) than without the intervention. If they paid less, they would be better off. A non-monetary concept of well-being is converted into a monetary equivalent. The difficulty is one of measurement; while you can ask a person directly in a public opinion survey how much they would be willing to pay for action, you can question the answer since you know that in reality they would not have to pay. In direct questioning (e.g. stated preference methods like *contingent valuation*) respondents tend to state much higher values than those they would be willing to pay in a real situation. In response to such problems, methods have been developed using market settings, such as eliciting willingness-to-pay values from real choices using experimental auctions.[14] These are auctions in which people reveal their preferences by spending money on different goods and products. These goods differ in their characteristics owing to policy intervention such as food irradiation or genetic modification. For example, after providing information about the adverse consequences of eating too much salt, one might observe the choice of participants in an experimental auction among substitute products with different salt levels. It is much harder to think of a relevant set of product attributes that could be used to evaluate obesity and its health consequences.

To avoid having to find WTP or WTA, a modification on the theme of *cost–benefit analysis* (CBA) is *cost–utility analysis* (CUA). This focuses on the 'utility' gained by those subject to the intervention measured through *quality adjusted life years* (QALYs) or *disability adjusted life years* (DALYs). These methods are now widely used in public health to account for utility, by recognizing that people value poor health less highly than good health, and interventions that make people feel better are valuable. Policy alternatives would be ranked according to their cost per QALY gained. Both QALYs and WTP are measures of utility, so how do QALY and WTP measures of utility relate to one another? The answer depends on how QALYs are measured; we proceed to address this issue now.

The aim of QALYs is to measure in a single figure the impact of an intervention that increases both life expectancy and the quality of life. Conceptually this is done by assuming that different states of ill health can be assessed in terms of the utility they provide relative to perfect health over a period of one year. For example, a case of food poisoning that caused five days of mild diarrhea might be unpleasant, but would be unlikely to reduce one's quality of life considered over a whole year by more than 1%. Let's call it 1%, in which case the person's QALY over the year would be 0.99. Thus, an intervention that prevented the case of food poisoning would yield 0.01 QALYs, though if it saved a million people from having food poisoning every year this would amount to 10,000 QALYs per year. If the intervention also saved 100 lives, total savings would be 10,100 QALYs per year. If such an intervention cost $100 million and an alternative investment of $100 million into, say, safer rail travel saved 500 QALYs per year, then the food poisoning intervention can be said to be more cost-effective. In principle all interventions should have the same cost per QALY gained. Otherwise a reallocation of resources from

---

[14] See Shogren et al. (1994, 1999, 2000); Hayes et al. (1995).

Table 3.1. The NICE EQ-5D quality adjusted life years valuation technique

Mobility

1. I have no problems in walking about
2. I have some problems in walking about
3. I am confined to bed

Self-care

1. I have no problems with self-care
2. I have some problems washing or dressing myself
3. I am unable to wash or dress myself

Usual activities (work, study, household, family, or leisure)

1. I have no problems performing my usual activities
2. I have some problems performing my usual activities
3. I am unable to perform my usual activities

Pain/discomfort

1. I have no pain or discomfort
2. I have moderate pain or discomfort
3. I have extreme pain or discomfort

Anxiety/depression

1. I am not anxious or depressed
2. I am moderately anxious or depressed
3. I am extremely anxious or depressed

high to low cost per QALY saved interventions could save more QALYs for the same total outlay. This is the principle underlying the decisions of the National Institute for Health and Clinical Excellence (NICE) in the UK. The institute is responsible for deciding whether new health interventions by the country's National Health Service (NHS), for example the use of a new drug, should be permitted. Given the limited resources of the NHS, not all new drugs can be afforded even if they improve health. NICE requires an estimate of the costs and quantification of the QALYs gained and has approved new interventions when the cost per QALY is below about £30,000 ($60,000).[15]

In the approach used by NICE, QALYs are measured using a validated questionnaire designed to elicit people's well-being in various conditions of ill health relative to perfect health. For example, a specific valuation technique, EQ-5D, is recommended by NICE in the UK and by authorities in the Netherlands, Norway, Italy, Hungary, Poland, Portugal, Canada, and New Zealand.[16] Health states are evaluated across five dimensions, each with three health states as in Table 3.1.

---

[15] This is not a hard-and-fast rule; some flexibility is allowed to take into account the degree of uncertainty, benefits to specific disadvantaged subgroups, and so forth.

[16] Szende et al. (2007).

People complete a questionnaire and give an evaluation of their overall well-being (between 0 and 1). A statistical analysis of a large survey has been used to estimate weights people attach to the various health states (these vary by country). Given the weights, which are publicly available in Szende et al. (2007), a risk assessment needs to specify the health benefits associated with a policy intervention in terms of the reduced number of people suffering each category of ill health in Table 3.1 to calculate the QALY gains. For example (purely hypothetically), if the average scores for diabetics from Table 3.1 is 1,2,2,2,2, they can be aggregated into a single score through the appropriate weights and compared with the average score of someone in perfect health. This makes it possible to estimate the relative quality of life. For example, one could estimate that a diabetic only has 50% of the quality of life of someone in perfect health. If obesity caused 1 million cases of diabetes, this would correspond to 0.5 million QALYs lost every year to diabetes.

This discussion suggests that the calculation of QALYs is straightforward and uncontentious, but this is not so. First, QALYs can be improved by discounting distant over proximate years of health saved. People value a year of good health now more highly than a year of good health in fifty years' time, so a policy to reduce, say, salmonella illness today might be valued more than an intervention to reduce obesity, which reduces risks of cancer, diabetes, and heart disease in the distant future. As discussed in Chapter 2 in relation to time discounting, the choice of discount rate is problematic. Something like 3% p.a. is typical for government projects, implying that €1 in one year's time is worth only 97 cents today and €1 in twenty years' time is worth only $1/(1.03)^{20} = 55$ cents now.

What about children? Is an intervention that protects young children more valuable because they have more years of life ahead or less because they can be *replaced* at low cost—and no money has so far been invested in their education and training? That the economist's perspective would ask such an unpleasant question does not make it any less relevant in a world of scarcity. The World Bank uses an approach which attaches the greatest value to 25-year-olds: money has been invested in their education and they have a full working life ahead of them.[17] Implicitly, this means that one is valuing only the social contribution of lives saved. But the approach is at odds with economists' notions of utility, which consider how much people will pay to save the lives of children relative to adults. Evidence suggests that parents rate their babies' lives as *more* valuable than their

---

[17] World Bank (1993).

own. For instance, parents often buy organic baby food although they do not eat organic food themselves.

In a world of rudimentary data, these issues may be academic. A simpler approach that avoids associating utility values to states of ill health is to look only at the life years (LYs) saved by an intervention (these can also be discounted). This approach ignores ill health and concentrates only on mortality, but may be acceptable if closely correlated with QALYs. Studies by Chapman et al. (2004) and Robberstad (2005) suggest that in over 80% of cases priorities associated with alternative policy interventions are unchanged when ranking by LYs or QALYs.[18]

Valuing the lives saved is a necessary part of any economic impact assessment of food policy. The most common approach is to calculate the value of a statistical life (VSL). The VSL reflects how much the representative person would pay to reduce the probability of death. While one might think that no one would give up their life for any amount of money, we make these risk–money trade-offs everyday, e.g. speeding in a car. People will pay to increase the *probability* of living longer, e.g. we pay for airbags and other safety features. Consider an example from Mason et al. (2006). Suppose an intervention affects 100,000 people and reduces the probability of death to each by 1 in 100,000. This implies that the intervention would save, statistically, one life. Suppose, further, on average each person was willing to pay $10 for this reduction in risk. The total value of the one life saved is $10*100,000 = $1 million. Actual figures used in the US and UK are typically between $3 million and $7 million.[19]

Problems arise when thinking how to measure the VSL and with interpreting its consequences for food policy. If rich people will pay more for food and health, for example, does this mean a rich person's life is more valuable than a poor one's? What is the implication for policies to reduce health inequalities? Should we value an extra year of life for a 70-year-old the same as for a 20-year-old? We do not delve deeply into these issues here. Rather we note that if the VSL is accepted as the value an average member of society places on life, if we divide by average life expectancy, L (about forty-five years remaining in a population of average age around 35), it is reasonable to assume that the value attached to each year is approximately VSL/L, or about $90,000 if VSL is $4 million (about the value used by the Department of Transport in the UK). This is a reasonable

---

[18] Chapman et al. (2004); Robberstad (2005).
[19] See Viscusi and Aldy (2003), who examine the VSL of over sixty studies in ten countries.

starting point for the valuation for a QALY, although it would be improved by discounting distant over proximate years saved.[20] The figure is higher than the implicit value of $60,000 placed on a QALY by NICE, but close enough not to cause alarm.

We summarize this section:

- Efficient resource allocation requires society to measure the costs and benefits of alternative interventions.

- Measuring costs is conceptually straightforward, though it may be challenging in practice to elicit from companies the true costs of complying with a regulation. Firms have an incentive to overstate the costs and an accounting procedure assumes that they will not alter their production or marketing processes or product formulations in response to the new incentives provided by the regulation. For example, front-of-pack nutrition labeling through a traffic light system may induce firms to reformulate their products to move from a red (unhealthy) signal to amber. However, other firms may use cheaper ingredients to move from, say, the healthy end of amber to the unhealthy end of amber since the signal to consumers would be unchanged. Such responses to incentives are hard to predict or measure through the usual survey methods used by regulators.

- Measuring benefits is problematic because interventions affect quality of life and life expectancy. Public health officials and economists have adopted a utility-based approach and implicit monetary valuation of a QALY.

- Economists would like to apply the monetary value of QALYs gained by an intervention, set it against the costs of the intervention, and assess whether benefits exceed costs to decide whether the intervention is worthwhile. The public health approach relies on cost–utility analysis as a rationing mechanism, but this does not reveal whether a policy intervention would pass a benefit–cost test.

- Economists are more concerned than public health professionals to distinguish private and social benefits when evaluating interventions. QALYs are measures of private benefits, as such they should be 'counted' when evaluating an intervention only to the extent that they reflect an increase in people's utility, which is not necessarily the case with interventions to reduce obesity.

---

[20] Fisher et al. (2005).

Ex Post Economic Evaluation of Policy Intervention

This chapter emphasizes how economists can make policy intervention more effective by evaluating the costs and benefits of obesity. But we have also pointed out that existing data are inadequate for rigorous assessment. While governments have increasingly required cost–benefit analysis prior to policy measures (ex ante analysis), interventions are inadequately monitored and assessed once the intervention has been completed (ex post analysis). This is important if one wants to learn, for future interventions, from how firms and consumers actually respond to incentives.

Economics cannot control the world like an experiment in a laboratory. In the lab, a researcher can create the counterfactual: the control for the road not taken. In the real world the experimental factor cannot be varied while holding everything else constant; nevertheless, the last decades have witnessed progress in bringing principles of the experimental approach to the policy evaluation scene, especially thanks to the econometric work of the 2000 Nobel Laureate James Heckman. Evaluating the impact of an intervention means looking into the difference between the actual outcome of the policy measure and what would have happened without the policy. Suppose the objective of evaluation is the impact of a national public information campaign on daily salt intake. A correct evaluation is not the measure of salt intake before and after the campaign, because salt intake might have been changed by other factors than the policy (e.g. price changes). A possible option would be to compare the salt intake of subjects reached by the information campaign relative to the intake of subjects not reached by the campaign. For example, one could compare residents in another part of the country (if such a regional experiment could be organized) or in another country. But again, other uncontrollable factors may differ between the two groups. When an experimental design is possible, the distinction is between the *treatment group* (the group which is reached by the intervention) and a *control group*, which should be similar to the treatment group in all characteristics but the exposure to intervention.

Economists call this *specifying the correct counterfactual*. Comparing the costs obese people impose on the health service to those of non-obese people requires one to hold constant all other factors influencing health costs. We want to compare two people who are identical in all respects except that one is obese. This has been referred to in the smoking literature as the 'non-smoking smoker', someone who has all the attributes of a smoker (attitudes, income, demographics, and social class) but does not smoke. The point is that obese people also tend to have lower incomes and lower education, and smoke and drink more. All associated factors might contribute to a person's health care costs, but comparing the health care costs of obese and non-obese people would attribute them all to obesity; this is a common mistake.

The problem in social science is finding an appropriate control group. Biases are likely because of differences in both observable characteristics (e.g. age, education level, prices, income, etc.) and, more importantly, in non-observable characteristics, like those due to selection bias. Selection bias arises because subjects in the treatment and control group differ in the starting conditions.

For example, if an information campaign aimed at reducing salt consumption is broadcast through TV advertising, heavy TV watchers are more exposed to the intervention. However, heavy TV watchers might also be more inclined to adverse health consequences for other reasons than consuming salt (for example, because of reduced physical activity). The control group also needs to include heavy TV watchers for a proper assessment of the health impact of the information campaign. Accounting for all sources of bias remains a challenge.[21]

Various methods have been devised to take account of self-selection bias,[22] in which a counterfactual group is built by selecting a set of people who match the intervention group with respect to a selection of variables. The success of the operation depends on whether the set of variables chosen is sufficient to eliminate systematic differences. The more complete the set of possible variables, the more expensive and time-consuming the experiment.

A modern econometric route to non-experimental ex post evaluation is the use of *difference-in-difference estimators*, also known as natural experiments. Two differences are computed: (1) the difference in the outcome variable for the treatment group, before and after the policy intervention; and (2) the difference in the outcome variable for the comparison group, before and after the intervention. The method is able to allow for dissimilar characteristics between the treatment and control group by assuming that these dissimilarities do not vary over time, so that by comparing the changes in outcomes between the two groups the actual policy impact is isolated. This method can be linked to the multivariate modeling approach by regressing the difference variable (before and after the

---

[21] Blundell and Costa Dias (2000).
[22] Heckman et al. (1997).

intervention) on a set of observable characteristics plus a dummy variable to distinguish between the intervention and control groups.

Endogeneity is a further problem in modeling (recall the case study in Box 2.2). People make choices for numerous variables simultaneously, for example, smoking, calorie intake, and exercise. The amount of exercise taken depends upon calorie intake and vice versa; in statistical terms, the variables are endogenously determined. Explaining obesity requires one to account for this endogeneity.[23] A model that attempts to explain obesity as a function of calorie intake and exercise while assuming that those two variables are exogenous would produce statistically biased estimates unless simultaneous equation estimation methods were used. Policy evaluations based on biased coefficient estimates would be misleading at best.

Among examples of evaluations and estimations dealing with non-experimental data, Morris (2007) accounts for endogeneity and exploits matching to find a significant impact of obesity on employment in the UK, while Tchernis et al. (2007) reverse previous evaluations of the impact of the US School Breakfast Program (SBP) and the National School Lunch Program (NSLP) after allowing for selection bias. Previous evaluations suggested that participation in the SBP was associated with an increase in children's weight (hence a negative impact of the program), while the NSLP was found to be unrelated to weight outcomes. Accounting for selection bias means acknowledging that overweight children are more likely to participate in the programs, hence affecting the final evaluation. After correcting for the bias, it was shown that the SBP is indeed an effective instrument to reduce children's weight, while the NSLP is detrimental.

In summary:

- It is useful to conduct ex post policy evaluation. Past experience can help us to understand the potential effectiveness of new policies.

- Since we cannot control the world like an experiment in a laboratory, other tools are needed. Modern econometrics provides these tools. Methods have been developed to avoid the biases inherent in any uncontrolled experiment, notably involving specifying the correct counterfactual, avoiding selection bias, and compensating for endogeneity.

- Data availability problems continue to restrict formal evaluation of past policy. This is due to the relative newness of obesity policy interventions and the difficulty in obtaining a time series of comparable data covering the pre- and post-intervention. Generating this data remains an important area for future research.

---

[23] See e.g. Rashad (2006).

Conclusion

Markets matter for health policy; markets work and markets fail. If markets fail, government intervention is beneficial; otherwise health-improving measures may be ineffective or they may end up worsening social welfare. To move from theory to practice, this chapter has provided further findings and guidance:

1. The costs of obesity can be internal to the market if they are borne by obese people themselves. For example, evidence suggests that obese people, especially women, have lower salaries and more difficulties in finding employment, and die younger. Obese people also suffer the health consequences of their decisions.

2. If we focus on external costs of obesity—costs imposed on others owing to private consumption decisions—society should focus on medical (direct) and employment (indirect) costs. Evidence suggests that medical costs of overweight and obesity may amount to 5% of health care costs in the US, which is 0.5% of GDP. Indirect costs associated with days off work are less precise and more controversial. Estimates suggest that they equal or exceed medical costs.

3. Private costs of obesity, those associated with ill health and premature death, have not been measured. Instead, quality adjusted life years, or QALYs, that attach a utility value to these conditions could be used. A QALY value of $60,000 is a useful benchmark to evaluate the benefits of a policy intervention designed to revamp diets, reduce obesity, and improve health. The value of the QALYs can be set against the costs of the intervention to determine if welfare improves.

4. From a social cost–benefit perspective, private benefits should be included when the intervention enables people to make more informed choices. They should be excluded when the intervention pushes people away from their preferred behavior; if, for example, they adopt a higher level of health at the expense of other goods and services, e.g. eating more than they should, or eating fast foods. Healthier is not necessarily happier. Here only the social benefits of intervention should be counted on the benefit side. In evaluating interventions it is important to be clear what costs should be counted and why.

5. Ex post evaluation of policies is important to learn lessons for the future, but difficult outside the arena of the controlled experiment. Modern econometric methods have shed light on how this may be achieved

but lack of data has made these methods difficult to use. This will change over time, and in Chapter 4 we provide examples of such procedures.

References

Allison, D. B., R. Zannolli, and K. M. V. Narayan (1999), 'The Direct Health Care Costs of Obesity in the United States', *American Journal of Public Health*, 89/8: 1194–9.

Baum, C. L., and W. F. Ford (2004), 'The Wage Effects of Obesity: A Longitudinal Study', *Health Economics*, 13/9: 885–99.

Bhattacharya, J., and M. K. Bundorf (2005), *The Incidence of the Healthcare Costs of Obesity*, NBER Working Papers 11303 (Cambridge, Mass.: National Bureau of Economic Research).

Blundell, R., and M. Costa Dias (2000), 'Evaluation Methods for Non-Experimental Data', *Fiscal Studies*, 21/4: 427–68.

Carpenter, C. S. (2006), 'The Effects of Employment Protection for Obese People', *Industrial Relations*, 45/3: 393–415.

Cawley, J. (2004), 'The Impact of Obesity on Wages', *Journal of Human Resources*, 39/2: 451–74.

Chapman, R. H., M. Berger, M. C. Weinstein, J. C. Weeks, S. Goldie, and P. J. Neumann (2004), 'When Does Quality-Adjusting Life-Years Matter in Cost-Effectiveness Analysis?', *Health Economics*, 13/5: 429–36.

Finkelstein, E. A., I. C. Fiebelkorn, and G. J. Wang (2003), 'National Medical Spending Attributable to Overweight and Obesity: How Much, and Who's Paying?', *Health Affairs*, 22/4: W219–W226.

—— C. J. Ruhm, and K. M. Kosa (2005), 'Economic Causes and Consequences of Obesity', *Annual Review of Public Health*, 26: 239–57.

Fisher, G., T. Kjellstrom, A. J. Woodward, S. Hales, I. Town, A. Sturman, S. Kingham, D. O'Dea, E. Wilton, and C. O'Fallon (2005), *Health and Air Pollution in New Zealand: Christchurch Pilot Study* (Wellington: Health Research Council, Ministry for the Environment, Ministry of Transport).

Garcia, J., and C. Quintana-Domeque (2007), 'Obesity, Employment and Wages in Europe', in K. Bolin and J. Cawley (eds), *The Economics of Obesity* (Amsterdam: Elsevier).

Hayes, D. J., J. F. Shogren, S. Y. Shin, and J. B. Kliebenstein (1995), 'Valuing Food Safety in Experimental Auction Markets', *American Journal of Agricultural Economics*, 77/1: 40–53.

Heckman, J. J., H. Ichimura, and P. E. Todd (1997), 'Matching as an Econometric Evaluation Estimator: Evidence from Evaluating a Job Training Programme', *Review of Economic Studies*, 64/4: 605–54.

McPherson, K., T. Marsh, and M. Brown (2007), *Tackling Obesities: Future Choices: Modeling Future Trends in Obesity and the Impact on Health* (London: Government Office for Science).

Mason, H., A. Marshall, M. Jones-Lee, and C. Donaldson (2006), *Estimating a Monetary Value of a QALY from Existing UK Values of Prevented Fatalities and Serious Injuries*, University of Birmingham, Department of Public Health and Epidemiology Reports RM03/JH13/CD.

Morris, S. (2007), 'The Impact of Obesity on Employment', *Labor Economics*, 14/3: 413–33.

National Audit Office (2001), *Tackling Obesity in England* (London: Her Majesty's Stationery Office).

Oliver, J. E. (2006), *Fat Politics: The Real Story behind America's Obesity Epidemic* (New York: Oxford University Press).

Pagán, J. A., and A. Dávila (1997), 'Obesity, Occupational Attainment, and Earnings', *Social Science Quarterly*, 78/3: 756–70.

Paraponaris, A., B. Saliba, and B. Ventelou (2005), 'Obesity, Weight Status and Employability: Empirical Evidence from a French National Survey', *Economics and Human Biology*, 3/2: 241–58.

Popkin, B. M., S. Kim, E. R. Rusev, S. Du, and C. Zizza (2006), 'Measuring the Full Economic Costs of Diet, Physical Activity and Obesity-Related Chronic Diseases', *Obesity Reviews*, 7/3: 271–93.

Rashad, I. (2006), 'Structural Estimation of Caloric Intake, Exercise, Smoking, and Obesity', *Quarterly Review of Economics and Finance*, 46/2: 268–83.

Robberstad, B. (2005), 'QALYs vs DALYs vs LYs Gained: What Are the Differences, and What Difference Do They Make for Health Care Priority Setting?', *Norsk Epidemiologi*, 15/2: 183–91.

Roglic, G., N. Unwin, P. H. Bennett, C. Mathers, J. Tuomilehto, S. Nag, V. Connolly, and H. King (2005), 'The Burden of Mortality Attributable to Diabetes: Realistic Estimates for the Year 2000', *Diabetes Care*, 28/9: 2130–5.

Shogren, J. F., S. Y. Shin, D. J. Hayes, and J. B. Kliebenstein (1994), 'Resolving Differences in Willingness-to-Pay and Willingness to Accept', *American Economic Review*, 84/1: 255–70.

—— J. A. Fox, D. J. Hayes, and J. Roosen (1999), 'Observed Choices for Food Safety in Retail, Survey, and Auction Markets', *American Journal of Agricultural Economics*, 81/5: 1192–9.

—— J. A. List, and D. J. Hayes (2000), 'Preference Learning in Consecutive Experimental Auctions', *American Journal of Agricultural Economics*, 82/4: 1016–21.

Szende, A., M. Oppe, and N. J. Devlin (2007), *EQ-5D Value Sets: Inventory, Comparative Review and User Guide* (Dordrecht: Springer).

Tchernis, R., D. L. Millimet, and M. Hussain (2007), *School Nutrition Programs and the Incidence of Childhood Obesity*, CAEPR Working Paper 2007–14.

Tucker, D. M. D., A. J. Palmer, W. J. Valentine, S. Roze, and J. A. Ray (2006), 'Counting the Costs of Overweight and Obesity: Modeling Clinical and Cost Outcomes', *Current Medical Research and Opinion*, 22/3: 575–86.

van Baal, P. H. M., J. J. Polder, G. A. de Wit, R. T. Hoogenveen, T. L. Feenstra, H. C. Boshuizen, P. M. Engelfriet, and W. B. Brouwer (2008), 'Lifetime Medical Costs of Obesity: Prevention not Cure for Increasing Health Expenditure', *PLoS Medicine*, 5/2: e29.

Viscusi, W. K., and J. E. Aldy (2003), 'The Value of a Statistical Life: A Critical Review of Market Estimates throughout the World', *Journal of Risk and Uncertainty*, 27/1: 5–76.

Wada, R., and E. Tekin (2007), *Body Composition and Wages*, NBER Working Papers 13595 (Cambridge, Mass.: National Bureau of Economic Research).

Wild, S., G. Roglic, A. Green, R. Sicree, and H. King (2004), 'Global Prevalence of Diabetes: Estimates for the Year 2000 and Projections for 2030', *Diabetes Care*, 27/5: 1047–53.

Wolf, A. M. (2002), 'Economic Outcomes of the Obese Patient', *Obesity Research*, 10: 58S–62S.

—— and G. A. Colditz (1998), 'Current Estimates of the Economic Cost of Obesity in the United States', *Obesity Research*, 6/2: 97–106.

World Bank (1993), *World Development Report 1993: Investing in Health* (New York: Oxford University Press).

4

Policy Intervention

Economics can help decide whether an intervention is sensible in principle, determine the data that should be collected for later evaluation, predict the outcome of the intervention, evaluate it ex ante against accepted criteria and evaluate it ex post against the same criteria. This chapter explores two broad areas of obesity policy intervention which we broadly define as *information measures* and *market intervention measures*. For information measures, we discuss the main objectives driving information campaigns, advertising regulations, nutritional education programs in schools, labeling rules, nutritional information on menus, and regulating health and nutrition claims (see Table 4.1).

For market intervention measures, we examine taxes on unhealthy nutrients, subsidies for healthy nutrients, regulating liability of food companies, food standards, facilitating access to shopping areas for disadvantaged categories, and regulating catering in schools, hospitals, etc. In the following sections we explore these policy interventions in more detail. We assess the evidence from the research literature about the effectiveness of each measure, and we highlight the additional data necessary to carry out a comprehensive policy evaluation.

Policies to counter obesity are recent, so they have rarely been evaluated formally and comprehensively. All too often a policy is declared effective if it changes people's attitudes or knowledge. But the next step—evaluating whether an intervention has changed people's consumption—is much harder; a comprehensive economic evaluation is rare. If the consumption response to a policy measure can be assessed, ex post evaluation is straightforward in principle. Ex post evaluation requires information on the direct and indirect effects of diet on health; and of their social valuation (QALYs, health care costs, etc., as discussed in Chapter 3). Such evaluations do not presently exist, though formal ex ante evaluation based on predicted

Table 4.1. Nutrition policy instruments classified by type of intervention

Policy instrument	Immediate objective[a]
Information measures	
Information campaigns	Increase consumer awareness
Advertising regulations	Limit/ban advertising of unhealthy foods (especially when targeted to children)
Nutritional education programs in schools	Increase awareness and knowledge of nutritional requirements and health consequences
Labeling rules	Promote informed choice by signposting healthy and unhealthy nutrients
Nutritional information on menus	Promote informed choice in eating-out situations (blamed as one of the most relevant factors)
Regulating health and nutrition claims	Define rules and monitor the use of nutrition and health claims in promoting and labeling food products
Market intervention measures	
Tax on unhealthy nutrients	Reduce consumption of unhealthy foods
Price subsidy for healthy nutrients	Increase consumption of healthy foods
Regulate liability of food companies	Monetize negative externalities of production/sale of unhealthy foods
Food standards	Setting nutritional standards for processed products to limit the access to unhealthy nutrients or promote consumption of beneficial nutrients
Facilitating access to shopping areas for disadvantaged categories	Address the issue of store dispersion in low-income areas by facilitating access to supermarkets for disadvantaged categories
Regulate catering in schools, hospitals, etc.	Contrast the tendency of allowing snack vending machines or fast foods in public places in exchange for private funding of activities
Funding epidemiological, behavioral, and clinical research	Improve supply, health care, knowledge

[a] The final objective of all interventions is to improve diets.

Source: Adapted from Mazzocchi and Traill (2005).

consumption changes are increasingly used to guide policymaking by the UK Food Standards Agency (FSA).[1]

In this chapter we explore examples of policies that have been introduced or proposed in a range of countries, though we make no claims that the examples are comprehensive. We also present what fragments of empirical evidence of effectiveness exist in the research literature and we complement this with the use of economic logic to suggest the probable effectiveness of interventions and hypothesize about unintended side-effects.

---

[1] For example, recent Regulatory Impact Assessments for folate fortification of flour and restrictions on advertising to children predicted gains in QALYs from the interventions and put a monetary value on these to calculate cost–benefit estimates.

The primary objective of information measures is to correct asymmetries and imperfect information to enable consumers to make better-informed choices. We discuss whether this is effective or has the anticipated outcomes, but we should note here that even were such interventions to result in everyone making perfectly informed choices, they would do so to maximize their own private welfare, and people would still choose to be overweight. This would not overcome problems of externalities, costs imposed by obese people on the rest of society through health care costs and lost productivity. To correct this market failure, economists would advocate that everyone pays a price that reflects the true social cost of their actions, not just the private costs. A fat tax is the most direct way to achieve this goal, though other interventions may indirectly achieve the same goal.

Information Measures

The *perfectly informed* consumer chooses his or her own diet to maximize his or her own satisfaction given their preferences, incomes, and the relative prices in the market. But if individual choice is based on incomplete or wrong information, government or third party intervention may be justified. More information on the diet–health relationship can cause a person to reassess the well-being associated with each choice option. Even with better information, however, consumers may still choose an unhealthy diet. Policymakers who promote information measures need to recognize and appreciate that this choice may be rational in a market setting.

We assume that the object of information (and education) from a government's perspective is to inform people better of health risks and the benefits of healthy eating. Information measures need to get their message across. Information on the risks of unhealthy eating targeted at someone unaware of the risks should improve their diet as they take the new risks into account, but targeted at someone who thought the risks were much higher, the information may lead to a downward revision of risks and the adoption of a less healthy diet.[2] We can see that information and education targeted to a person who is already well educated and informed would have no impact on their diet. As Kuchler et al. (2005a) state, 'the sheer volume of media coverage devoted to diet and weight makes it difficult to

---

[2] People believe food additives and pesticide residues at levels in food for sale in shops in developed countries are harmful, whereas these have been passed as safe by domestic and international food safety regulators.

believe that Americans are unaware of the relationship between a healthful diet and obesity'. The authors quote surveys that show most American consumers to be aware of health problems associated with certain nutrients and able to discriminate among foods on the basis of fat, fiber, and cholesterol. The same knowledge is likely present in adults in most middle- and high-income countries.

The relationship between information and education (which improves critical faculties and enables people more accurately to assess 'true' relationships between diet, obesity, and health, and healthy eating behavior) is, a priori, indeterminate.

Economists refer to the welfare loss from poor information as the *cost of ignorance*.[3] It is possible to show that welfare is maximized when the information people act on is accurate, so those who underestimate or overestimate risks should gain welfare from better information. We know of only one study that attempts to measure the cost of ignorance in relation to diet choice (Teisl et al. 2001). This study shows that labeling can increase individual welfare *even if it produces no health benefit*. The authors examined choice between 'healthy' and 'unhealthy' foods in the same product category, such as between semi-skimmed and full-fat milk. The welfare gains arise from people being able to choose what they prefer rather than from any implied health benefits. For mayonnaise and salad dressing, the authors found that labeling *reduced* the share of the healthy product purchased—presumably because 'low fat' products are perceived as being less tasty. In this particular example, information increases individual welfare because it enables better-informed choice, but it probably reduces health.

Policy evaluators need to understand how much consumers (in aggregate or by socio-economic group) respond to information by changing their diets. As we shall see, the evidence is limited and sometimes conflicting. Assessing the impact of information measures is complicated because the effects of information policies are not immediate and are not long-lasting because people can forget: in statistical terms, the lag structure of consumer response to information is complex.

Public Information Campaigns (Social Marketing)

The principle behind *social marketing*, as Halpern et al. (2004) argue, is that government cannot deliver policy outcomes (including diet and exercise) to a disengaged and passive public. Greater personal responsibility enables

---

[3] Foster and Just (1989).

117

society to function with a less intrusive state and can deliver public goods more cheaply.[4] Social marketing is the application of commercial marketing techniques such as consumer-oriented market research, segmentation, targeting, and other elements of the marketing mix to social issues with the objective of improving individual and social welfare (rather than to make profit).[5] Gordon et al. (2006) have carried out a systematic review into the effectiveness of thirty-one social marketing interventions in relation to nutrition. They conclude that these have been effective in increasing knowledge and self-efficacy, and in changing attitudes, but less effective in changing blood pressure, BMI, and cholesterol levels.

Gordon et al. argue that this is because of the long timescale needed to influence these outcomes. They believe that the funding of social marketing should be measured in decades rather than years. But neither clinical nor economic studies have provided sound evidence that public information leads to improved consumer behavior. Still, public information campaigns raise little opposition, so they remain popular. Examples include the 5-a-day fruit and vegetable campaigns in several countries and the campaign to cut salt consumption by the UK FSA.

Evaluations of social marketing campaigns have major limitations, however, since they do not address any interaction with market forces (see Box 4.1), For example, when the UK Department of Health piloted the 5-a-day program based on local initiatives,[6] the key findings were positive:

- a half-portion higher intake in the intervention group compared to the control group;
- an overall positive effect on people with the lowest intakes;
- an increased awareness; 17% increase in the intervention group who correctly reported that 5-a-day was the optimal fruit and vegetable intake compared to 8% in the control group.

The pilot study (over twelve months) was not limited to public information campaigns and also included action to improve access to fruit and vegetables by retailers and food cooperatives, and targeted promotional activities in the community and by primary health care professionals.

An impact assessment by the European Commission[7] claims that information measures can improve knowledge and change attitudes about diet

---

[4] Halpern et al. (2004: 7).

[5] Stead et al. (2007).

[6] Department of Health, *Five-a-Day Community Pilot Initiatives: Key Findings*, <http://www.5aday.nhs.uk/original/locally/documents/Pilot_key_findings.pdf>.

[7] European Commission, *Impact Assessment Report accompanying the White Paper 'A Strategy for Europe on Nutrition, Overweight and Obesity Related Health Issues'*, Commission Staff Working

and exercise. The document cites an extensive review carried out by the University of Teesside and published by the National Institute for Health and Clinical Excellence.[8] Based on twenty studies selected for their scientific rigor (from sixty-six total), the main conclusions of the review are:

- *Impact on diet.* Evidence suggest that promotional campaigns including media interventions can increase awareness, among children as well as adults, of what constitutes a healthy diet and *may* improve dietary intakes.

- *Impact on exercise.* Evidence is unclear whether media interventions can influence participation in physical activity. Studies suggest that interventions may be more successful if they target motivated subgroups; promotional campaigns including media interventions can improve knowledge, attitudes, and awareness of physical activity.

- *Impact on body weight.* Limited evidence exists that a multi-component intervention, including a public health media campaign, can have a beneficial effect on weight management among people of higher social status; the effectiveness of promotional campaigns focusing on education alone are unclear.

In short, the balance of evidence on the effectiveness of information campaigns and social marketing is that they raise awareness but do not affect behavior.[9] The public sector has lacked marketing skill, so today its use of advertising professionals is commonplace. Another reason is the time decay of information, which calls for a continuing rather than one-off campaign, not always possible given the uncertain nature of funding.[10] Furthermore, research shows that when risks are well known (e.g. smoking risks, but also with obesity), public campaigns are ineffective in changing behavior.[11]

Document, SEC(2007) 706/2, <http://ec.europa.eu/health/ph_determinants/life_style/nutrition/documents/nutrition_impact_en.pdf>.

[8] National Institute for Health and Clinical Excellence (2007), *Obesity: The Prevention, Identification, Assessment and Management of Overweight and Obesity in Adults and Children*, app. 5, pp. 1052–1127, <http://www.nice.org.uk/guidance/index.jsp?action=download&o=38284>.

[9] See Seiders and Petty (2004) and references therein.

[10] An interesting direction has been taken in France, where the Public Health Law requires food companies to choose whether to accompany adverts with health information or to pay a financial contribution equal to 1.5% of their promotion and advertising expenditure to support state nutritional information campaigns.

[11] Rindfleisch and Crockett (1999).

Box 4.1. Case study: Impact of the 5-a-day information campaign on demand and consumption

The setting is the adoption of an information policy by the UK Department of Health, which launched a 5-a-day campaign in March 2003 to increase fruit and vegetable consumption toward the target of five portions per day. The program consisted of a set of interventions, including a School Fruit Scheme and a communications program, plus concerted actions with the supply sector. The timing of the campaign launch creates a natural experiment as it was launched in March, which corresponds to the end of the fiscal year. Since the UK Expenditure and Food Survey gives data on fruit and vegetable consumption by fiscal years, we can use the 2002/3 data set to benchmark the consumption situation before the campaign and 2003/4 to assess the effects of the first twelve months of the campaign. We rely on actual data for this case study, although we simplify the economic and quantitative modeling issues. The temptation and the practice in public health evaluations is to compare the levels of consumption before and after the campaign, which in this case would involve comparing data from the 2002/3 survey with those of 2003/4 and attributing changes to the information change. This implies looking at consumption: the final equilibrium outcome, rather than the effects on demand. The economic approach is to evaluate the change in consumption *after* allowing for the effect of changing prices and incomes. This allows us to isolate the effects of information on demand.

Table 4.2 shows the consumption levels for different income quartiles, only considering households residing in England. As expected, the poorest households show the lowest consumption levels. They also pay the lowest unit value, which represents the price they chose to pay, among those available on the market.[12]

The richest households consume almost twice as much fruit and vegetables as those in the lowest quartile and they also pay higher unit values. Following the 5-a-day campaign, we observe a significant drop in purchases for low-income households (almost −11%), And small changes for other income quartiles. Unit values increase for all income quartiles, with an average rise of about 4.2%. Considering actual market prices, government statistics show over the same period a nominal increase of 2.4% for fruit and 8.3% for vegetables at the retail level. Considering real prices (compared to the general food price index), vegetables showed a 6.7% increase and fruit also became more expensive (+0.9%). In the year following the launch of the 5-a-day campaign, fruit and vegetables became more expensive compared to other foods.

In summary, if one evaluates the effect of the 5-a-day campaign by considering Table 4.2, one can conclude that information had no systematic impact on consumers. But eliciting the true impact of the campaign requires that one understands what would have happened to purchases in 2003/4 if prices and incomes had remained the same as in 2002/3.

To keep this example straightforward, assume that fruit and vegetable purchases are affected by changing prices (relative to other foods) and incomes. Consider a

---

[12] The unit value is the ratio between expenditure and quantity purchased; it reflects the actual price paid by consumers. A higher unit value might reflect either an increase in price or the choice of a product with a higher quality (and price).

Table 4.2. Fruit and vegetable expenditure in England and unit values[a] before and after the 5-a-day campaign

Income quartile	April 2002/March 2003		April 2003/March 2004		Change (%)	
	Quantity purchased (kg per household per week)	Unit value (£ per kg)	Quantity purchased (kg per household per week)	Unit value (£ per Kg)	Quantity	Unit value
Lowest	4.35	0.153	3.88	0.166	−10.75	9.03
Medium–low	5.66	0.164	5.79	0.174	2.45	5.84
Medium–high	6.70	0.176	6.84	0.178	2.20	0.62
Highest	8.40	0.187	8.29	0.194	−1.31	3.24
TOTAL	6.36	0.171	6.26	0.178	−1.51	4.25

[a] Unit value is calculated as expenditure divided by quantity purchased.

demand function in which fruit and vegetable purchases for each household in the sample are determined by the relative price of fruit and vegetables to other foods and household income:

$$Q_{FV} = f(P_{FV}/P_{OF}, I)$$

where Q_{FV} is the quantity purchased of fruit and vegetables, P_{FV} is the price of fruit and vegetables, P_{OF} is the price of other foods, and I is the household income. We consider a multiplicative functional form, which has the desirable property that it can be transformed into a linear one using logarithms and the estimated coefficients are price and income elasticities, a useful measure in economics. The price (income) elasticity (explained in Chapter 2) measures the percentage change in consumption determined by a 1% increase in price (income). We have the demand equation:

$$\log Q_{FV} = \alpha + \varepsilon_P \log(P_{FV}/P_{OF}) + \varepsilon_I \log(I).$$

This means that the purchased quantity depends on prices, incomes, and elasticities.

If we estimate this relationship on data for the period 2002/3, we obtain values for the intercept and the elasticities as shown in Table 4.3. The price elasticity ε_P shows that a 1% increase in the price of fruit and vegetables relative to the price of other foods leads to a decrease of −0.34% in the amount purchased. The income elasticity is also low since a 1% increase in income implies an increase of 0.35% in purchased quantities. The intercept α is a measure of the average level of household purchases when all other variables are zero. This model is assumed to explain fruit and vegetable purchase decisions in 2002/3.

Table 4.3. Fruit and vegetable demand model on 2002/3 data: elasticities

	Coefficient	Standard error
α	6.832	0.089
ε_y	−0.34	0.017
ε_I	0.35	0.015

In the year following the launch of the 5-a-day campaign, prices and incomes both change. If we apply the model to price and income data for 2003/4 and simulate the purchases of each household, assuming price and income are the influential factors, we compute the purchased quantities that we would have recorded in 2003/4 *without the 5-a-day campaign*. These quantities are computed for each family as follows:

$$\log \hat{Q}_{FV}^{2003/4} = 6.832 - 0.34 \log (P_{FV}/P_{OF}) + 0.35 \log (I)$$

in which the prices P_{FV} and P_{OF} and the income I are taken from the 2003/4 data set. The same data set also provides the quantities *actually* purchased by each of the households. Since these actual quantities also reflect the effects of the 5-a-day campaign, we elicit the impact of the intervention after eliminating the effects of varying prices and incomes. Table 4.4 illustrates the results, which differ significantly from those of Table 4.2. For all income quartiles, a major increase in purchases emerges. The intervention has had positive effects, but these were in practice offset by price increases.

Table 4.4. Impact of the 5-a-day campaign

Income quartile	Without 5-a-day (model based estimates) (kg per household per week)	With 5-a-day (actual data) (kg per household per week)	Change (%)
Lowest	3.21	3.88	20.82
Medium–low	4.24	5.79	36.53
Medium–high	5.23	6.84	30.83
Highest	6.82	8.29	21.57
TOTAL	4.93	6.26	27.09

What happened with 5-a-day information?

Although our model is stripped down to basics to be illustrative, it demonstrates why economics matters when planning and evaluating interventions in the health and nutrition area: the impact of the campaign has been mitigated by the market. According to FAO data, the UK produces about 3 million tons of fruit and vegetables per year, while total consumption is more than twice that level (approximately 7 million tons). Most of the demand for fruit and vegetables is met by imports (in 2004 the UK imported about 8.4 million tons of fruit and vegetables versus less than 1.2 million tons exported). The internal supply of fruit and vegetables is likely to be rigid in the short term and excess demand is met by more expensive imports. The final market outcome is an equilibrium which results from demand meeting supply. Informed consumers may desire to buy more fruit and vegetables, but supply is unavailable to meet additional demand, especially in the short term. If importing more fruit and vegetables is more expensive, the main effect of information is a price increase. Actually, fruit and (especially) vegetables show noticeable price increases in the aftermath of the campaign. If the final objective of the policy was the increase in fruit and vegetable consumption and not the profits of the fruit and vegetable sector, an information policy was ineffective, at least in the short term. A similar campaign in Western Australia, named 'Go for 2 & 5', was found to be effective, with a significant increase in fruit and vegetable servings per day across the population.[13] Australia is self-sufficient in both fruit and vegetables and domestic supply exceeds consumption.

Advertising Controls

Advertising is an action by the private sector to promote a product and increase company revenue, especially in markets with a high concentration of firms. The point is often made that firms spend huge amounts advertising foods, generally unhealthy ones (advertising expenditure is highest for soft drinks, breakfast cereals, confectionery, snack foods, and fast foods; see e.g. Skinner et al. 2005), and they wouldn't do it if it was ineffective. The argument goes that banning advertising would lead to less consumption of unhealthy foods. Firms counter that advertising encourages brand switching rather than category expansion (e.g. Pepsi advertising encourages people to switch from Coca-Cola to Pepsi rather than to increase overall soft drink consumption). The key questions for economic analysis are the usual ones. First, would advertising controls promote healthier diets and improved health? Second, would the benefits exceed the costs?

The costs associated with banning private sector advertising are nebulous to capture. Much depends on market competition, which defines how firms interact with one another, and on the impact of advertising on overall demand (as opposed to brand share). Suppose advertising only affects brand share for a product. Using a game-theoretic approach, there would be contexts in which advertising was harmful to the firms in the market—the so-called prisoners' dilemma, in which everyone has to do it because everyone else does, even though all firms' profits could be enhanced by colluding among themselves not to advertise or by legislation banning advertising. But in other contexts, it could be argued that advertising and innovation go hand in hand and banning advertising would restrain product development, innovation, and economic growth.

What would be the cost to consumers of an advertising ban? A ban on heavily advertised foods would reduce the demand for advertising time and space and result in a fall in the cost of advertising and in advertising

---

[13] Pollard et al. (2007).

revenue to advertising companies and TV stations, magazines, and the Internet. These media are mostly funded by advertising. Less revenue would reduce media output or quality, or a search for alternative means of financing them, and higher prices for magazines, subscription television, etc. To our knowledge, no research has calculated these costs of an advertising ban.

Can advertising regulations, like banning junk food adverts in children's TV programs, improve diets? This issue has long been investigated, with mixed answers. The UK FSA commissioned a systematic review of scientific evidence on the extent and impact of food promotion to children.[14] The reviewers conclude, based on the fifty-one scientific articles, that an effect exists on children's brand awareness, preferences, requests to parents, and purchase behavior, both at brand and at category level, but the evidence of a link with modified consumption patterns is still weak and inconsistent.[15] Researchers maintain that the relationship between advertising and obesity is not scientifically substantiated.[16] For example, a food advertising ban to children in Quebec since 1980 has not resulted in lower childhood obesity prevalence than in other Canadian provinces, and a similar ban in Sweden since the early 1990s has not reduced obesity prevalence.[17] The evidence is clearer on the link between television viewing and obesity, but this can also be attributed to lack of physical activity.[18]

Two alternative forms of advertising regulation exist:[19] self-regulation and public regulation.[20] Self-regulation requires the food industry to develop voluntary codes and guidelines, like the Children's Advertising Review Unit (CARU)[21] in the US, funded and supported by major advertisers and with a main remit for food advertising.[22] Similar self-regulation efforts exist in other countries.[23] CARU monitors advertising to children and handles complaints (which can be submitted online through the web site). They also open 'cases' when issues arise, and address problems with

---

[14] Hastings et al. (2003); a US-specific review can be found in Story and French (2004).

[15] Coon and Tucker (2002).

[16] See Zywicki et al. (2004) and references therein.

[17] Ashton (2004).

[18] Viner and Cole (2005).

[19] Armstrong and Brucks (1988).

[20] For a detailed review of regulations, monitoring, and self-regulations in the area of advertising to children, with a close focus on food adverts, see Hawkes (2004).

[21] <http://www.caru.org>; see also Armstrong (1984).

[22] <http://www.cbbb.org/initiative>.

[23] See Hawkes (2004, table 5) for a detailed list of statutory and self-regulatory measures in advertising to children.

the advertisers, who may voluntarily adjust or withdraw the advert. CARU may decide to refer the case to a government agency. In 2004, for instance, CARU opened a case against Unilever,[24] because of a food advert (and product label) referring to 'Real Fruit Juice Pops', whereas the product only contained 30% fruit juice. Unilever agreed to modify the claim into 'with 30% Fruit Juice'. Figures over thirty years (from 1974 to 2003)[25] show that CARU has handled about 1,100 cases, 150 of them on food. This means that either the industry behaves ethically or CARU is ineffective. We say this considering that in 2000 the average American child watched an estimated 40,000 food commercials.[26]

The alternative to self-regulation is to place explicit restrictions on advertising, such as the content, duration, and scheduling of the adverts, up to a complete ban on certain types of advert.[27] In Sweden and Norway advertising to children is prohibited. Norway does not permit commercial sponsorship of children's TV programs, advertising during children's programs, or TV advertising directed to children under 12.[28] Proposals to restrict advertising exist in other countries,[29] but food industry opposition has made these politically difficult to implement. In the US, for example, the Federal Trade Commission's attempts to ban or regulate advertising to children (like the 'Food Rule' of the late 1970s) have been limited by political decisions because of conflicts with the First Amendment (freedom of speech).[30] Most existing regulations are targeted to avoid misleading information and to substantiate nutrition and health claims. In France the Public Health Law requires food companies to accompany adverts with health information or, failing that, to pay a financial contribution equal to 1.5% of their promotion and advertising expenditure to support the state nutritional information campaign.

In terms of improving information, researchers have argued that regulating advertising might have adverse effects. This argument is based on the evaluation of the US Nutrition Labeling and Education Act (NLEA)

---

[24] <http://www.caru.org/news/2004/unilever.asp>.

[25] NARC (2004).

[26] Cawley (2006) and references therein.

[27] A review of the performances and legal aspect of the two alternative routes (self-regulated or public control bodies) can be found in Alderman et al. (2007).

[28] Prevention Institute (2002).

[29] Hawkes (2004) lists among others Australia, Brazil, France, Germany, India, Ireland, Italy, Malaysia, New Zealand, Poland, and the United Kingdom; a list of countries with advertising regulations is shown in table 3 of the article. Petty (1997) compares US and EU advertising regulations.

[30] See Pappalardo and Ringold (2000); Dunkelberger and Taylor (1993); Sheehan (2003); or Petty (1997).

introduced in 1990, which set standards for health claims including those used in advertising. While the regulation was supposed to improve information available to consumers, regulatory standards reduce advertising in relation to health claims for those products that are less profitable, while more profitable (and possibly unhealthy) products continue to be advertised, especially those that do not rely on health claims.[31] It was found that the regulation brought a decline in advertising for healthy foods like fruit and vegetables, while advertising of snack foods was not affected by the NLEA.

The case against regulating advertising is based on the so-called 'unfolding' theory of advertising.[32] Since the NLEA obliges producers who wish to make a health claim to highlight undesirable and desirable nutritional characteristics, producers decide not to advertise. Instead, if they were permitted to advertise only the positive characteristics in an environment allowing for competitive advertising, other producers would pinpoint the product deficiencies of competitors and overall information to consumers would 'unfold'. This line of reasoning is valid when substitutes in the same category may be superior in a few product attributes. This logic fails when substitute products are homogeneous in terms of good and bad characteristics.

It remains difficult to link regulations on food advertising to actual outcomes in terms of improved nutrition or reduced obesity. But indications on the effectiveness of advertising bans can be drawn by looking at tobacco, though even here the message is mixed. A study on the impact of advertising bans[33] in twenty-two OECD countries estimated that the overall effect of promotion and advertising increased tobacco consumption by around 6–7%. In contrast, a study[34] on the impact of advertising bans on youth smoking in developing countries, which have been targeted by the industry, concluded that partial advertising bans (e.g. on advertising before, say, 9 p.m.) did not affect youth behavior in a significant manner.[35] Others have argued that less advertising increased consumption because it lowered firms' costs and so enabled them to lower prices.[36]

---

[31] Ippolito and Pappalardo (2002).
[32] Ippolito and Pappalardo (2002).
[33] Saffer and Chaloupka (2000).
[34] Nelson (2003a).
[35] Bans on advertising were more likely to stop people taking up the habit than persuading existing smokers to give up. To the extent that obesity results from addiction or habit formation, this finding may be of relevance.
[36] See e.g. Nelson (2003b).

We conclude that although advertising bans, particularly on unhealthy foods to children, are becoming common, and appear publicly acceptable, their economic impact remains poorly understood. Consensus has been reached on the impact of advertising on awareness, but research linking this to eating behavior and obesity is incomplete. As well as the impact of advertising on diets, a proper economic cost–benefit evaluation would need to consider the possibility that banning or limiting advertising may have the paradoxical effect of preventing complete information from unfolding.

Nutritional Labeling

Nutrition labels are a primary source of information on food products and have been the subject of policy interventions around the world. Research has focused on consumer use of label information and on the search for the most effective label content.

Although nutrition labels may be viewed as a precondition for informed choice, studies note how complex nutrition labels, those requiring more thought on the part of consumers, could lead to misusing or ignoring labels. For example, sugar and saturated fats exist in almost all foods and their recommended intakes are expressed in terms of percentage of total calorie intake. Computing this value for the overall diet from label information on individual foods demands knowledge but also time and a willingness to use scarce time. For economists, these are transaction costs that can be significant for a busy consumer (see Chapter 2). When transaction costs are too high, the consumer may choose not to use the label or to exploit only part of the information. Regulations imposing even more detailed nutritional requirements on labels may be ineffective.

In most countries nutrition labeling of processed food is voluntary. The US is an exception and the EU is planning to make nutritional labeling compulsory. In general, regulation specifies the format labeling should take if manufacturers decide to use nutritional labels. This has resulted in multiple formats internationally despite the best efforts of the *Codex Alimentarius*, which has established international nutrition labeling guidelines.

In the US nutrition labeling rules were set under the Nutrition Labeling and Education Act (NLEA), introduced in 1990. A precise set of rules on the format of nutrition labels was delivered in 1993. This makes it possible to provide an evaluation of the economic impact of the NLEA, accounting for additional costs implied by the regulation (administration, testing, design, and print of labels—if exporting to countries with different require-ments—and monitoring) and the economic benefits, including improved nutrition. The first evaluations conflicted.[37] Some researchers have argued for high benefits[38] and others[39] claimed that costs were much greater than the benefits. One cost–benefit analysis[40] estimated the total costs of NLEA to be about $2 billion (as of 1996), while long-term benefits could be evaluated in the range of $100 billion. These major disparities in evalu-ation are due to prior assumptions, for example about the rate of mislead-ing claims prior to NLEA, and a robust economic assessment is difficult, especially when claims refer to uncertain diet–health relationships.[41]

A later study[42] supports the view that the social benefits of labeling outweigh the costs. The research concludes that consumers read labels and alter their purchase decisions, and that producers have responded to the incentives provided by labels by introducing new, healthier formula-tions such as low-fat foods to improve the nutritional profile of their labels. That said, they also calculate that nutrition labeling has had a minimal impact on the overall rise in obesity. An interesting evaluation is provided in Variyam and Cawley (2006), who look at the impact of mandatory labeling on obesity using a difference-in-difference method to account for existing trends (see Chapter 3). This study finds a significant impact of labeling on weight, but only for non-Hispanic white females. The total monetary benefit in terms of reduced cost of illness was esti-mated at about $166 billion (1991 dollars) over a twenty-year period. Recent evaluations[43] have found a clear benefit to the subgroup of people motivated to improve their diet but with limited knowledge.

It is interesting to note that labeling seems to attract more interest in avoiding 'bad' nutrients than promoting 'good' ones. For example,[44] infor-mation on fats has an impact on consumer assessment of health risks, but information on fiber does not. This matches up with experimental findings on the demand for foods, in which negative information has a more power-ful impact than positive information (see, for instance, Fox et al. 2002).

In Europe people have debated the merits of simplifying labels. A front-of-pack traffic light system has been proposed by the FSA in the UK. Under this scheme, red, amber, and green signposts for each nutrient highlight a decreasing degree of conflict with dietary recommendations.[45] This

---

[37] See Pappalardo (1996) and references therein.   [38] Silvergale and Hill (1996).
[39] Petruccelli (1996).   [40] Silvergale (1996).   [41] Pappalardo (1996).
[42] Golan et al. (2001).
[43] See Balasubramanian and Cole (2002) and references therein.
[44] Garretson and Burton (2000).
[45] Bussell (2005).

signposting system raised a question about *oversimplification*. Oversimplification could be misleading and nutritionists confute theories of 'bad' and 'good' foods in favor of 'bad' and 'good' diets.[46] The largest UK supermarket chain, Tesco, has rejected the traffic light system in favor of a label indicating guideline daily amounts (GDA, the proportion of recommended daily intake made up by consuming a portion of the food in question).[47] But research by the FSA shows that people understand and support the traffic light system, and they prefer it to GDA. Both of the schemes are currently voluntary in the UK, while the European Commission has adopted a proposal which favors GDA, but allows for alternative labeling schemes at national level, like the FSA traffic lights. The competing systems are new, so it is too early to judge their effectiveness in changing behavior. Grunert and Wills (2007) review the existing research on how labels affect behavior and how the new signposting strategies were tested through consumer panels. According to the few studies run by supermarkets that look at actual purchasing behavior, traffic lights and other simplified labels like GDAs do not lead consumers to avoid unhealthy foods; they moderate their consumption. Again, evidence points to substitution to a healthier option within the same product category. But, as Grunert and Willis point out, scientific evidence has looked at perceptions, liking, and (overreported) purchase intentions, while there is little insight on the behavioral impact of simplified labels. We know that gaps exist between declared intentions and actual behaviors.

Sweden has been a leader in simplified labels. The Swedes introduced a *keyhole* symbol, which manufacturers can voluntarily use to signpost foods with low fat or high fiber, in categories in which there may be both healthy and unhealthy alternatives (for example, the symbol cannot be used for fruit).[48] Evidence suggests that consumers exploit the simplified message, but not less educated subgroups of the population (which coincide with higher-risk groups).[49]

We conclude that the balance of evidence is that consumers do make use of nutrition labels and they do have an impact on diet choices. The little research on costs and benefits also suggests this to be a beneficial intervention, though much of the research is based on survey responses; real responses using data generated in the marketplace are preferable.

---

[46] Krebs (2004).
[47] F. Lawrence, 'Tesco Rejects Traffic Light Food Labelling', *The Guardian*, 10 Mar. 2006 (accessible online on <http://www.guardian.co.uk>).
[48] Bruce (2000).   [49] Larsson et al. (1999).

We remind readers of the study discussed in the section 'Information Measures' above; the welfare loss from poor information is referred to as the *cost of ignorance*[50] and a study employing this approach shows that labeling can increase individual welfare *even if it produces no health benefit*[51] by enabling people to make better-informed choices corresponding to their personal preferences and economic circumstances.

Consumers balance additional information with their tastes: there is substantial variation across different food categories,[52] and signposting triggers substitution within the same category. The implementation of mandatory regulations should rely on accurate evaluations of transaction costs for both firms and consumers to avoid imposing a cost on society which is not reflected by a beneficial outcome. In calculating the benefits of labeling, account should be taken of the response to labels by firms who change the composition of their products to obtain a more attractive label. In this respect, companies have criticized the signpost approach, arguing that no realistic reformulation would move products like chocolate or cheese from a red to amber label for fat content. The system removes the incentive for reformulation and doesn't allow consumers who want to continue eating chocolate and cheese to substitute a healthier product in the category.

Eating Out and Nutrition Facts on Menus

More meals are now taken away from home (about half of total food expenditure in the US). This has led to the suggestion that nutrition facts should be shown on restaurant menus, similar to product labels. But labeling of unprocessed foods and meals taken outside the home (including takeaways) has proven difficult. No country has introduced such requirements. One British study[53] suggests that 'lower-fat' information for a meal in a restaurant was associated with it being chosen less frequently. Presumably, as with Teisl et al.'s (2001) nutrition labeling example, customers did not expect the low-fat meal to taste as good, and health was not a major factor in their decision of what to eat in a restaurant context.

In assessing the benefits of intervention, the issues are similar to nutrition labeling of processed products. The most difficult empirical obstacle is

---

[50] Foster and Just (1989).   [51] Teisl et al. (2001).
[52] See Grunert and Wills (2007).
[53] Stubenitsky et al. (2000), quoted in Variyam (2004).

to calculate the effect of labeling on the nutrition content of consumers' overall diets. As with the labeling of processed foods, change may come about either through consumers altering their behavior or through restaurants responding to incentives. People could choose healthier options on the menu or eat in restaurants providing healthier meals, or food service outlets could respond to incentives and change their recipes to improve the nutrient profile of their meals so that their labels are more 'attractive' (in terms of the nutrition information they provide). The labels may encourage a new and advantageous form of non-price competition among restaurants. Neither effect can be identified over a short period of time using an intervention study to observe what meals consumers choose when they are labeled or not. Longer-term time series of actual consumption of all foods, with and without the intervention, is necessary. The evidence on the actual impact of nutrition information on menus in terms of energy and nutrient intakes is weak,[54] both in the US[55] and in the UK.[56] In contrast, evidence suggests that consumers are unaware of the high levels of unhealthy nutrients in menu items[57] and provision of information goes in the direction of allowing informed choice. Increased awareness has prompted a market solution to the problem: the number of restaurants willing to provide nutritional information on menus is increasing[58] even in the absence of legal requirements.

This last observation runs counter to one argument against nutritional labeling in catering outlets: that the costs are prohibitive. The prohibitive costs argument could be valid for small restaurants that have neither the capacity for nutritional testing nor the desire to standardize their offerings in terms of ingredients or portion sizes. Compulsory legislation would accelerate the process of structural change: the displacement of small independent restaurants by large chains. It is doubtful that this is what consumers want.

Health and Nutrition Claims

Health and nutrition claims are popular in the food industry. They act as marketing tools. But if used inconsistently, they can mislead consumers, inducing uninformed and unhealthy food choice.[59] This holds when health claims are made in promotional material rather than labels;

---

[54] Finkelstein et al. (2004) and references therein.   [55] Variyam (2004).
[56] Kral et al. (2002); Stubenitsky et al. (2000).   [57] Burton et al. (2006).
[58] Wootan and Osborn (2006).   [59] See e.g. Hartmann et al. (2005).

promotional materials and claims on labels are often regulated by different bodies (for example, in the UK the FSA is responsible for label information, the Advertising Standards Authority for the accuracy of advertising material; in the US the respective bodies are the Food and Drug Administration and the Federal Trade Commission). Misinformation plays a large role in the Internet era. The American Dietetic Association has reported[60] that the top three sources of nutrition information for consumers are television, magazines, and newspapers; 48% of consumers cite television as a leading source against 1% recorded for dietitians and nutritionists, 11% for doctors, and 12% for books. The report notes that the estimated number of consumers looking for health information rose from 70 million in 1999 to 100 million in 2000. The problem is that the quality of information disseminated through the mass media or the Internet shows a great deal of variation in terms of quality and reliability, leading to a rising degree of confusion among consumers.

Sellers make health claims about their product—that they produce health benefits or reduce disease risk; for example, that the product lowers the level of cholesterol in the blood or is good for the heart. The regulatory challenge is to balance these claims against the fact that relationships for specific nutrients and health are still up for scientific debate and considerable disagreement still exists about the degree of proof required for a claim to be permitted. Different countries have demanded different levels of proof; a country can favor a liberal approach to encourage innovation and perhaps the competitiveness of their industries. A country can have a tough burden of proof, as demanding as for the introduction of a new drug. The European Commission adopted a regulation on the use of nutrition and health claims for foods in 2006.[61] This regulation produces EU-wide rules aimed at ensuring that claims are clear, accurate, and substantiated, much like the NLEA regulation in the US.

From our perspective of evaluating the net benefits of legislation, one benefit, in addition to any change in consumer purchase behavior, is the strong incentive it provides for private research in nutrition and for product innovation toward healthier alternatives. Furthermore, regulating health claims can be seen as a tool for ensuring fair competition and promoting innovation, since only substantiated health claims can be used to promote products.

---

[60] See American Dietetic Association (2002).
[61] <http://ec.europa.eu/food/food/labelingnutrition/claims/index_en.htm>.

Health claims can trigger undesirable effects too. One study found that health claims: (*a*) reduce the actual search for nutrition information; (*b*) lead consumers to weight the health claim more than nutrition facts on the label; and (*c*) induce a positive perception (not based on evidence) that other attributes of the product also have a positive health effect.[62] Another study[63] showed that the 'low-fat' claim induced consumers to eat larger quantities and that the reduction in fats may not correspond to a reduction in energy-density, which is what matters.[64]

Nutritional Education

Nutrition education is a wide and varied field, ranging from nutrition in schools to setting up ad hoc courses for adults. In the US programs successful in changing behavior (but not necessarily body weight) stressed family involvement, self-assessment activities, intensive instruction times, and coordination with interventions in the school environment.[65] In Finland nutrition education is a part of home economics courses all school students study for at least one year.[66]

Evidence[67] exists suggesting that more nutritional knowledge is associated with healthier behavior, but the relationship is not straightforward. A well-conducted statistical analysis of the impact of nutrition knowledge on BMI was run on data from Taiwan.[68] This study included questions on participants' knowledge of the link between obesity and various health outcomes. The researchers looked beyond the mean BMI to examine (through quantile regression techniques) the impact of knowledge on BMI for those in different BMI quantiles of the population (holding constant other factors that influence obesity such as age and ethnicity). They found that low-weight men and those moderately overweight were not influenced by health knowledge. But obese men did respond to health knowledge: they are significantly less obese than they otherwise would be. For females the relationship is not statistically significantly different from zero at any percentile. The results, particularly for men, highlight how education and knowledge most likely affect those who are most at risk. Also, from the empirical analysis standpoint, they highlight the dangers of analyzing responses at the mean: the relationship between *mean* BMI and nutrition knowledge is not statistically significant. There is no reason to expect people

---

[62] Roe et al. (1999).   [63] Miller et al. (1998).   [64] Swinburn et al. (2004).
[65] See the review by French (2005: 111–15).   [66] Roos et al. (2002).
[67] See e.g. Dallongeville et al. (2001).   [68] Kan and Tsai (2004).

who are not overweight to change their eating behavior in response to information that tells them that being overweight is bad for them.

Policy Evidence for Information Measures

The large—albeit insufficient—body of evidence suggests a few principles on the effectiveness of information policies and their evaluation.

1. We make the point that better education and information enables people to make better-informed choices and this is a precondition for welfare maximization. But if uninformed or uneducated people overestimate the risks of unhealthy diets they may respond by eating less healthily once informed and educated. There is no a priori hypothesis to specify which direction the response would be. Economists do not find it surprising that most researchers find weak empirical relationships between information, education, and diets.

2. Information is valuable to people because it enables them to make informed choices, even though it may not improve their diets.

3. Information measures are intended to enable people to make private decisions that maximize their individual welfare. If, as we suggested in Chapter 3, the problem with obesity is the externality by which medical and productivity costs are imposed by the obese on the rest of society, these measures will not help. Most people do not consider social welfare when making private decisions.

4. We note a recurring theme: words do not seem to match up with deeds. When surveyed, consumers say they are responsive to an intervention. But when aggregate data are observed and examined in detail, consumers' actions indicate that the *actual behavioral change* in the marketplace is much less marked. This is not a message limited to information measures but is much broader.

5. It is desirable to examine responses to interventions by obesity quantiles rather than estimate a mean response. For example, one might expect that information on the health risk of obesity affects those most at risk; that is, overweight and obese persons more affected than under- or normal-weight ones.

6. It is important when evaluating interventions that account is taken of market forces. If supply is rigid and markets saturated, higher demand leads to higher prices rather than higher consumption, which might worsen health inequalities.

7. It is important to consider firms' responses to regulation. Regulations can provide incentive for firms to change their behavior in a desirable direction in advertising, nutrition labeling, and health claims. But do they? And what are the unintended consequences of these regulations, for example on research and development? Policy evaluation should attempt to predict such changes.

Market Intervention Measures

Nutrition information, education, and social marketing constitute the largest portion of the budget for controlling obesity. Economists, however, have argued for more direct measures that could have a larger impact on behavior and health, and address the externality caused by obesity: obese people impose costs on the remainder of society through health care and lost production.

In particular, economists have proposed taxing foods expected to cause people to become overweight, such as confectionery, salted snacks, and foods high in fat or sugar. Alternatively, a subsidy could be given to the consumption of healthy foods, e.g. fruit and vegetables. These options have been called *fat taxes* and *thin subsidies*. The idea of taxes on unhealthy products or price support for healthy products has sparked an intense economic and political debate. We discuss the reasons why. An alternative way to internalize the obesity externality is to make firms legally liable for the health damages they cause, similar to food safety. We examine the literature in this area.

We also look at other policies that affect consumption through the market, even if diet and health were not their primary focus. The most notable example is agricultural policy, which has often been blamed for subsidizing farmers and thereby contributing to overeating. We investigate the validity of that argument. Other measures considered in this section include those that target diets by influencing the availability of food on the market, through the composition of processed foods and catering in the public sector.

Taxes and Subsidies

Economists have long explored the role of taxes and subsidies to address market failures. If an externality exists because the price people pay for food does not reflect its cost to society, a tax or subsidy intended to align private and social costs and prices is the appropriate theoretical tool. We examine whether it would be effective or have any undesirable side-effects. Although such fiscal measures can be used to lead to healthier diets, the impact of a tax or subsidy is undesirable if taxes on foods have undesirable distributional effects, i.e. impose disproportionate costs on the poor or generate disproportionate benefits to the rich.

The direct economic effect of a tax is that consumers lose welfare because they pay higher prices and consume less of the taxed goods than they would at market prices. Producers also lose revenue because they sell less and at a lower price. These losses are balanced by a gain in tax revenue and a gain in public health (the objective of the intervention). The difference between the losses to consumers and producers and the gains in tax revenue is known in economics as the 'deadweight loss' of the policy measure. To show the policy to be worthwhile, it is necessary to show that the benefits of reduced consumption of unhealthy foods outweigh the deadweight losses. It is also necessary to show that the distributional consequences of the tax are acceptable between rich and poor consumers, between regions, and between ethnic groups, but also between large and small firms.

For subsidies the situation is reversed: consumers and producers both gain, but the taxpayer loses because the subsidy must be paid. The difference between gains and losses is also known as the deadweight loss and must again be justified by the value of the gains in public health. One can imagine a simultaneous fat tax and thin subsidy, in which tax revenues finance the subsidy. Such an intervention encompasses two deadweight losses, two public health gains, and complex distributional consequences, in terms of both the distribution of financial consequences and the distribution of public health benefits.

As we discussed in Chapter 1, lower-income consumers are observed to be more obese on average and eat more foods considered unhealthy. They are also, because of their low incomes, more responsive to prices: their price elasticities are higher than those of wealthier consumers. This implies that they would bear a greater share of the tax burden and receive a lower share of the subsidy. But because they respond most to fiscal incentives, they would adjust their consumption more than the rich and gain most in terms of reduced health risks; the *health* benefits of taxation might be *progressive* even though the *economic* effects are regressive.[69]

---

[69] There is even the possibility of the paradoxical situation: by further reducing the income of poor households, a tax could lead to an increased demand for cheaper energy-dense foods; see Clark and Levedhal (2006).

The 'fat tax'[70] concept has been dismissed as ineffective because wealthy consumers are unresponsive to food prices; and regressive because poor consumers spend the largest share of their incomes on food, particularly 'cheap' energy-dense food; and unfair because the tax also falls on people who are not obese. One response to the first criticism is that previous studies have investigated low-level taxes at value added tax (VAT) rates, currently 17.5%. It is accepted that cigarette taxes have been effective[71] and they are applied in countries at much higher levels, as are taxes on alcohol. The evidence suggests that people respond to large incentives.

Mytton et al. (2007) investigated extending VAT (a form of sales tax) to certain categories of food. As alternatives they examined taxing the main sources of dietary fat, taxing foods using a wider nutrient-based definition of unhealthy, and taxing foods to achieve the best health outcome (the latter by 'judicious' trial and error). They employ own- and cross-price elasticities for foods from the existing literature and combine the implied consumption effects of the tax regimes with data from the literature showing the effects of intake of different fatty acids on cholesterol levels, and the impact of this and salt intake on the annual numbers of stroke, ischemic heart disease, and coronary heart disease deaths. They conclude that small health benefits can be achieved, but unexpected results are possible; for example, they find that taxing saturated fats results in increased salt intake and higher mortality overall. The study has the limitations that it refers only to foods consumed in the home, whereas meals outside the home are known to be more calorie-dense.

Leicester and Windmeijer (2004) examine the differential burden of the tax on rich and poor, but they do so assuming that the tax induces no change in food consumption: their estimate of the tax burden can be seen as an upper limit because people are not allowed the opportunity to respond to changed prices by switching to less highly taxed products. The authors calculate that the poorest 2% of the population would pay seven times as much *as a proportion of their incomes* as the richest 2%.

Chouinard et al. (2007) use US data and estimate a 'complete' (with all appropriate constraints imposed) set of elasticities and cross-price elasticities for fourteen dairy products (disaggregated to include 1% milk, 2% milk, whole milk, cheese, butter, etc.). They simulate a tax, proportional to fat content, of 10%. This reduces overall dairy fat intake by less than 1%.

---

[70] The term has been coined because unhealthy eating has been most commonly associated with excess fat intake. We would propose to generalize the concept to allow the possibility of also taxing calories, sugars, snacks, salt, or whatever is most effective and practicable.
[71] Goel and Nelson (2006).

They also look at the distributional burden and find that the burden (again as a percentage of income) is ten times larger for a family living on $20,000 per year than for one on $100,000.

Set against these findings, a recent study of Danish consumers considers a tax on saturated fats, a tax on sugar, and subsidies on fibers as well as revenue-neutral combinations of these fiscal instruments (Smed et al. 2007). These authors also estimate a set of demand elasticities and permit them to vary over six age groups and five social class groups because lower income/social class groups are known to be more responsive/elastic to price changes than higher income/social class groups. They find that a modestly sized revenue-neutral combination of taxes on saturated fats and sugars combined with a subsidy on fibers reduces saturated-fat consumption substantially, particularly in the two lowest social class groups. Sugar consumption is reduced by a smaller amount but by most in the three lowest social class groups;[72] fiber consumption rises substantially in all social class groups. This is achieved at the same time that the lower social class groups experience a fall in total food expenditure. The authors also conclude that a tax on nutrients is much more effective at bringing about desired changes in nutrient intakes than a tax on specific foods (through VAT, for example).

Cash et al. (2005) estimate that a 1% price subsidy on all fruit and vegetables could prevent nearly 9,700 cases of heart disease per year in the United States. They calculate that the cost of such policy intervention in terms of expenditure per life saved, on average $1.29 million, is below the common evaluations of the value of statistical life (see Chapter 3), which suggests that the thin subsidy would be beneficial for society.

Marshall (2000) looks at how increasing VAT affects ischemic heart disease. He considers raising VAT to 17.5% for foods that are the main sources of saturated fats. Marshall estimates a reduction in ischemic heart disease of between 1.8% and 2.6%; this would avoid about 1,000 premature deaths per year in Britain. This study reflects on a parallel tax increase: how the price differential between unleaded and leaded petrol affected car manufacturer behavior, arguing that a 10% gap induced an adjustment of supply and an increase in production of cars that could use the cheaper unleaded fuel. This is similar to the hypothesis that an increase in the price of energy triggers more innovation in energy-efficient technologies, which would lower the risks of climate change. This comparison raises

---

[72] There are five social classes in total. There are perverse results for the top social class.

the question: are fat and cholesterol the leaded fuel of food products and could a tax accelerate the transition to a healthier food supply?

Pragmatically, authorities may introduce taxes on unhealthy products to raise revenue for other nutrition policy interventions.[73] A tax on soft drinks in Arkansas of about 2 cents per can generates revenue of $40 million per year. Economists have estimated that taxes on soft drinks and confectionery throughout the US generate about $1 billion per year.[74] This money could be 'ring-fenced' to finance, for example, nutrition information and education policies.

A possible fiscal instrument which has received no attention would be aimed at affecting food composition through a tax on food manufacturers' use of unhealthy ingredients. These are substitutable in the manufacturing process, so a change in relative prices could persuade manufacturers to change their recipes. For example, people argue that saturated fat has become a cheap by-product of the dairy industry because consumers have moved from full-fat milk and butter to semi-skimmed milk and margarine. Dairy fat has become cheap, so manufacturers use a lot of cream in processed foods. If cream were taxed as an ingredient, its use would decrease. As always, there would be other repercussions: surplus dairy fat from rich countries would be exported to poor countries, causing them more ill health; and farmers may receive lower prices for their milk. Even if the tax is imposed on manufacturers, the price increase would be transmitted to farmers and consumers.

As far as we are aware, such a policy has never been introduced or discussed. We believe that it is a measure deserving attention, but evaluation would have to consider the various repercussions mentioned.

We conclude that there is growing interest in the use of fiscal measures to improve diets and make the prices people pay for foods reflect their true social costs. There is also a growing body of research which suggests that judicious selection of the targets of taxes and subsidies can overcome criticisms of their being regressive and ineffective. We view this as an important avenue for further economic research which may lead, in future, to real policy implementation.

Farm Policy, Income Subsidies, and Diets

Both in Europe and in the US, policymakers and the public continue to debate the relationship between diets and policy interventions outside the

---

[73] Kuchler et al. (2005*b*).   [74] Jacobson and Brownell (2000).

nutrition area, notably agricultural price support and the Food Stamp Program to support poor households. In Europe people ask whether the Common Agricultural Policy (CAP) is undercutting nutrition policy with its subsidies for dairying and sugar beet production. Experts in the public health area[75] have argued that subsidies to farmers lead to overproduction, encouraging overconsumption, especially for dairy products and sugar because these products are much more subsidized than fruit and vegetables.

But a proper consideration of economics and markets leads to the opposite conclusion. Farm price support in Europe is transferred to a large extent to consumer prices. As Ritson (1998) notes, there are two impacts on nutrition: through the overall cost of food, and through relative prices. Both effects suggest that the CAP is beneficial to healthy eating. Without it, food prices in Europe would be much lower than they are, leading to a boost in demand and further increase in energy intake. Furthermore, Ritson (1991) has shown that the CAP encourages healthy eating by operating like a fat tax; it raises the prices of dairy products and sugar.[76] Alston (2007) estimates that an elimination of farm support in the US would decrease sugar prices by about 15% against 5% for fruit and vegetables.[77] In Finland, before 1995 and EU membership, the state's support kept down the price of high saturated-fat dairy products, but since 1995 margarine and reduced-fat spread prices have fallen relative to butter[78] and this has contributed to a significant reduction in saturated-fat intake.

The US Food Stamp Program has also been blamed for increased obesity rates,[79] as recipients seem to consume more energy-dense foods than their non-eligible counterparts. But evidence is mixed and weak,[80] and the gap in body weight between participants and eligible non-participants has shrunk over time.[81] Overall, economists are skeptical about arguments that existing price support policies and food subsidies cause obesity.

POLICY INTERVENTIONS IN THE FOOD CHAIN

People blame the food industry for the obesity epidemic.[82] They argue that market power has directed choices away from healthy foods toward unhealthy foods and propose direct control of operations within the market. Much of the debate among commentators on market intervention and food policy divides down familiar exaggerated Right–Left lines. The Right trusts that the capitalist system works best with minimal regulation and

---

[75] Schafer-Elinder (2003, 2004); Leather (1996); von Haartman (1996); Lobstein (2002).
[76] Ritson (1991).   [77] See also Alston et al. (2006).   [78] Prattala (2003).
[79] See e.g. Chen et al. (2005).   [80] Hofferth and Curtin (2005); Kaushal (2007).
[81] Ver Ploeg et al. (2007).   [82] See e.g. Tillotson (2004) and references therein.

argues that regulatory zeal stifles innovation and thereby reduces its benefits. The Left think the present system is too lax and allows firms to exploit consumers by selling unhealthy food that kills people and trying to expand markets by duping and addicting unsophisticated consumers, notably children and the less well educated. This view demands much tighter regulation. Across countries, different political philosophies have developed different regulatory systems (e.g. the cooperative Nordic approach versus the more untrammeled capitalist Anglo-Saxon approach).

An open question we address in this section is the evidence for and against market power in the food industry and whether this is a justification for direct regulation of the market for food. If market power is affecting competition to provide healthy food, this would also be a market failure and intervention may be warranted. Competition generates gains to society by providing firms with incentives to produce efficiently, thereby lowering costs; and by innovating and selling goods that are of superior or different quality. An innovation need not produce a higher-quality good to be successful; it may be enough that some consumers prefer the new product. Consumers have different preferences: strong cheese versus mild; sweet and sour Chinese ready meal versus chicken and cashew; Ben and Jerry's ice cream versus Häagen-Dazs. Consumers also like variety. If the last ready meal was sweet and sour, next time one might choose chicken and cashew or Italian, Indian, Thai. In response, firms differentiate their offerings, selling goods that may vary according to a large number of characteristics including quality, price, flavor, environmental friendliness (organic, animal friendly, fair trade), and nutritional value. Farmers, food retailers, and restaurants differentiate themselves in a similar manner. People having new ideas and putting them into practice is what makes competition work; it works both by rewarding success and by punishing failure. But we know that firms in concentrated markets may face less competition to lower prices and innovate.

A firm may also be 'too' successful and drive all of its competitors out of business or buy them. Monopolizing the market enables the firm to charge an 'unfairly'[83] high price to consumers in the knowledge that it has no or few competitors to undercut it. The principles of social optimality discussed in Chapter 2 require perfect information, many market agents, and the absence of barriers to entry, so that firms are not price setters, but price takers. Market power is not limited to monopoly (one single firm), because

---

[83] Economists would not use the term 'unfair', but what is meant is an ability to charge a price for a good that exceeds its marginal cost of production.

in markets with few suppliers firms have discretion over the prices they charge. Antitrust laws do not require 100% market share before they consider that a firm has monopoly power; the figure is nearer 50%.

Market power allows firms to increase profits at the expense of consumers, by charging higher prices than those of perfect competition, but we saw in Chapter 2 that prices in food markets have followed a downward trend owing to technological advances. Of course, one may always argue that prices would have been even lower if conditions were more competitive, but if so, lower prices would have encouraged more consumption and more obesity. More relevant is price discrimination, which is segmenting the market and offering similar goods at different prices to different consumers, according to their willingness to pay. Firms may charge higher prices for healthy foods because people are willing to pay more for them.

It has been argued that prices are too low in fast food restaurants, but the fast food industry is one of the most concentrated. McDonald's controls almost half of the US market; the four main companies control 85% of the market.[84] Low prices cannot be imputed to imperfect competition, but rather to economies of scale. The same may be said of the high levels of concentration in food retailing. Nowadays[85] people are beginning to argue that food has become too cheap.

A related criticism is that supermarkets have driven small shops out of business; this is correct. But it has been argued that this has created 'food deserts', a scarcity of retail shops in poor areas at accessible distance and higher prices, particularly for fresh fruit and vegetables. This issue has received much attention in the public health literature[86] but the consensus is that such food deserts do not exist. Even in poor urban areas disadvantaged consumers have access to affordable healthy foods.

In addition to measures aimed to control market power, governments have several options to influence delivery of foods through the food chain. Most of these operate through measures to influence availability. For example, parents would favor prohibition on vending machines selling junk foods in schools. Few people question regulations requiring fortification of refined cereals (that have had their natural minerals and vitamins removed during refinement), but setting standards for the amount of fat or

---

[84] See Jargon (2006); Duecy (2006); and sales data from <http://www.technomic.com>.

[85] At the end of 2007. The subsequent food price spikes have put a stop, temporary or otherwise, to such suggestions.

[86] Food deserts have a dedicated web site with an up-to-date reference list, <http://www.fooddeserts.org>. On the date we visited the web site (26 Feb. 2008), 135 studies were listed.

sugar or salt in food is deemed interventionist—and an intrusion into personal liberty.

But the 'soft' policy of entering into a dialogue with industry to persuade it to cut back on these ingredients is deemed acceptable. It is becoming an essential component of nutrition actions in countries, starting with Finland's North Karelia Project,[87] and now extending to more libertarian countries like the UK. It is presumed that consumers are unaware of the levels of these nutrients in the foods they buy, so reformulation would have no negative impact on consumer welfare but would have a positive impact on health. The intervention is cheap for government, and firms may respond positively for the sake of their corporate image. When consumers are unaware of the ingredients in foods they consume (e.g. whether the fat in a processed food is saturated or contains high levels of trans fats), one may argue there are no obvious losers. But firms choose 'unhealthy' over 'healthy' ingredients for reasons of cost or taste. Recipe modification would either cost more or develop products that taste worse, so there would be a cost to consumers.

Interventions and Evidence on Food Availability in Schools and the Workforce

Concern about childhood obesity and the relationship between child and adult obesity has led people to call for restrictions on the supply of unhealthy food made available to children in schools and the provision of healthier meals to schools. The main targets are school meals and vending machines in schools that are loaded with unhealthy snacks and soft drinks, but in most countries interventions, if any, are recent.[88]

In Finland free school lunches have been served at comprehensives, upper secondary schools, and vocational institutes since the 1940s–1950s.[89] University students have also received subsidized meals since 1979. Menus are drawn up in schools and municipalities and lunches should meet a third of daily nutritional requirements. In Norway the custom is for almost everyone, including schoolchildren, to take a packed lunch, so there have been no policies targeted at school catering. This highlights the culture-specific nature of food behavior and the need for policies to be culture-specific: as usual, one size does not fit all.

---

[87] See e.g. Puska (2002).   [88] See French et al. (2003); Story et al. (2006).
[89] Roos et al. (2002).

The UK has been at the forefront in the privatization of the provision of school meals. Contracts go to the lowest bidder with no nutritional constraints imposed,[90] resulting in the average school meal costing 35 pence (less than 70 cents). The government has been shamed by a campaign by the celebrity chef Jamie Oliver to take the provision of nutritious school meals more seriously. In March 2005 the Education Secretary, Ruth Kelly, announced that at least 50 pence per pupil should be spent on food ingredients every day. She said, 'This new investment will transform what is offered to children and teenagers in our schools so that high-quality healthy food is on every child's plate.'[91] It is too early to assess the dietary consequences of this 'radical' move, but there have been reports that children have rejected healthy school meals in favor of packed lunches that contain potato chips (crisps) and chocolate.

As a separate action in the UK, part of its 5-a-day fruit and vegetable promotion scheme gives a free piece of fruit or vegetable every school day to primary school children. It is reported, based on pilot study evaluations, that the scheme results in children and their families increasing fruit consumption at home. In France free fruit distribution in schools has been evaluated through a pilot study of four regions: between 2003 and 2004 the percentage of schoolchildren consuming at least five portions of fruit a day rose from 27% to 35% in nursery schools and from 39% to 46% in high schools.[92]

In the United States much of the legislative authority over school meals and vending machines is under state control and, according to the National Conference of State Legislatures, in 2005 seventeen US states had enacted legislation over vending machines in schools.[93] Oliver (2006), however, says that much of the legislation imposes restrictions that are more apparent than real: limits are being imposed on certain types of school (not secondary) and at certain times of day.

Japan is interesting, having had standards on school food in force since 1954. Recall that Japan has the lowest obesity rate among OECD countries. The standards set strict limits on calories from fat in meals, as well as

---

[90] The 2001 nutritional standards for secondary schools given by the Department for Education and Skills (DfES) do require that at least two items from a number of food groups (such as starchy foods, dairy products, protein sources, fruit and vegetables) should be *available* every day (our italics). Nothing then to stop the children *choosing* sausage, beans and chips every day (http://www.dfes.gov.uk/schoollunches/secondary.shtml).

[91] DfES press release, 30 Mar. 2005, <http://www.dfes.gov.uk/pns/DisplayPN.cgi?pn_id= 2005_0044>. The DfES is revising the standards for school meals to reduce the fat, salt, and sugar content and to increase consumption of fruit and vegetables.

[92] Cresif (2004).   [93] <http://www.ncsl.org/programs/health/vending.htm>.

banning vending machines and restricting students from eating or buying food, drinks, or chewing gum while at school or while traveling between school and home.[94] In France a law envisaged in the National Nutrition Health Plan banned vending machines in schools from 2005.

These representative actions, in principle, make sense. Children tend to buy things that are available, particularly snacks and soft drinks, mainly because the time cost of buying and eating them is minimal. If it is made more difficult to obtain junk food, the benefits disappear and, one would expect, children cannot be bothered to make the effort to buy it. They eat the healthier food if the alternative is to go hungry, waiting until after school to buy junk. But we would need data on the impact of the interventions on children's consumption, and, to be able to assess the cost–benefit of the intervention, we would need to know how much the purchase of junk food in schools contributes to childhood food consumption and obesity. On the latter issue there is no information, although Oliver is skeptical as to how much blame for rising child obesity levels can be placed at the doors of schools. On the issue of the impact on consumption in schools, there is limited information.

The Finnish Nutrition Report for 2003 finds that although school canteens promote recommended food choices, and most schoolchildren eat a main course in the school canteen, half supplement it with something else, most commonly soft drinks and sweets.[95] The overall outcome might still be an improvement on what they would have eaten, even for those who supplement their lunches with junk food.

The American National School Lunch Program, within which 75% of American schoolchildren take their lunches, contributes to obesity: compared to children who eat a packed lunch, those who take a school lunch consume an additional 40–120 calories per day at lunch, and no fewer calories during the rest of the day.[96] This is an argument against providing unhealthy school meals, not an argument against school meals themselves. The data used by Whitmore Schanzenbach (2005) found that these children obtained a third of their daily calories from the school lunch, suggesting that the school meal is quantitatively important enough for healthier provision to make a significant contribution to diet quality if not quantity.

Collins and McCarthy (2005) investigate the determinants of consumption of certain 'junk' foods (or, as they describe them in the marketing

[94] Dalmeny et al. (2004).
[95] Finnish Nutrition Report 2003, <http://www.ktl.fi>.
[96] Whitmore Schanzenbach (2005).

vernacular, 'top-shelf' foods) by schoolchildren in Ireland. They employ the theory of planned behavior, developed in the psychology literature, to relate a person's planned behavior to their attitudes to the object in question, social norms, and behavioral controls. The behavior in question was purchase of junk foods (e.g. chips, burgers, confectionery, and carbonated soft drinks) during the school day (including travel to and from school). Survey data were collected on female adolescents' attitudes to these products (did they like them?), behavioral controls imposed by guardians (were they given pocket money?), and by schools (were they allowed to buy these products during the school day?), and social norms such as the importance attached to slimness by their peers. Their results suggest that school policy which restricts access to junk foods can reduce consumption during the school day, though they do not report by how much or its importance in relation to overall calorie intake.

In the US schools have entered into contracts with fast food and soft drink companies. School administrators have argued against a ban on vending machines because they are reliant on the income to make up for shortfalls in school funding:[97] school activities are paid for by junk food; 96% of American High Schools had vending machines in 2000 (though fewer at schools catering for lower age levels).[98] An important policy question is whether this in itself increases overall consumption (and obesity) or if children buy food at school that they would otherwise buy elsewhere, in which case the schools might as well take a share of the proceeds.

A careful study by Anderson and Butcher (2004) at a county level found first that variables representing financial pressure on schools, such as accountability regulations, population growth pressure, and the share of finances coming from public sources are good predictors of whether schools make junk foods available, allow various forms of food and drink advertising and promotion, and enter into exclusive agreements (pouring contracts). They observed that a 10% increase in the proportion of schools in a county that make junk food available to their students is associated with a nearly 1% increase in students' BMI.[99] Most interestingly, among children with at least one obese parent, the same increase in the proportion of schools allowing junk food increased obesity by more than 2%, whereas children with two normal-weight parents showed no BMI increase. This supports the view that policy should focus on those who are

---

[97] Oliver (2006).   [98] Anderson and Butcher (2004).
[99] Allowing advertising has no effect.

'vulnerable'. It raises the question of whether policies targeted at entire populations are fair to those who are not 'vulnerable'. The distribution of costs and benefits of a policy intervention can be important, along with the total.

To summarize, debates about freedom to choose an unhealthy lifestyle are put to one side when it comes to children. It is difficult to separate influences of parents, the environment in general, and the school-specific environment to evaluate the impact of school interventions on children's food consumption, but what limited analysis there has been suggests that the school environment is important, at least for those pupils who, for one reason or another, are at risk of weight gain. It also seems that there is an important cultural component to the sorts of interventions that are acceptable, and desirable. It is unlikely that the Japanese or Korean approaches, which emphasize traditional foods inside and outside schools, or the more moderate Scandinavian interventions would be acceptable in the more libertarian United States or UK. Strong food traditions in countries like France and Italy may also have a protective effect: if children's upbringing before attending school sets in concrete preferences that lead them, once at school, to *prefer* not to eat junk food and soft drinks, then they may be less at risk of obesity. But rising rates of adult and child obesity in these countries suggest that this might be an optimistic view in the long run.

Among adults, as far as we know, only Finland has intervened to influence diets through the provision of healthy meals. In Finland mass catering is said to play a key role in nutrition policy. Mass catering might have taught the Finns to eat vegetables.[100] Most women in Finland work, and catering at workplaces is usual. Workplace meal provision has been included in trade union agreements with both the public and private sectors since 1976, and advisory nutritional guidelines for such lunches have been issued since the 1970s. These are said to be followed, especially in the public sector. In Finland adults who eat lunch in staff canteens do eat more vegetables, and also fish and boiled potatoes.[101]

Liability under Law

Several lawsuits against US fast food chains are on hold pending appeal. The lawsuits claim that fast food companies were selling foods that made people fat, were addictive, and were served in too large portions. The legal

[100] Roos et al. (2002).   [101] Roos et al. (2002).

case is built around misleading advertising and lack of information about risks. Legal liability rules regulate how much of the financial responsibility for product failures should be borne by suppliers compared to consumers.[102] For example, if a product failure causes $1,000 damage to a consumer, there are two polar cases: strict and no liability. Strict liability imposes all costs on the supplier, and no liability imposes all costs on the victim (the consumer). A third rule is the negligence rule, which depends on whether reasonable precautions were taken by the supplier and on the basis of such evaluation allocates the monetary damage between the supplier and the consumer.

Economists have studied legal liability regimes in areas other than obesity; the results can be transferred to our problem. Economics needs to answer a difficult question: which liability rule is more efficient to prevent damage? Obesity is not a product failure and the link between the outcome and the 'injurer' is not straightforward. Consider the *Pelman* v. *McDonald's* case,[103] for example. Here an obese consumer who suffered diabetes sued the fast food company, on the grounds of misinformation, for encouragement to buy larger meals without stressing the side-effects. The judge dismissed the case because it was impossible to demonstrate McDonald's exclusive liability. Furthermore, law is not expected to intervene in the consequence of a consumer's bad decisions when the danger is 'open and obvious'.[104] Such lawsuits prompted the US House of Representatives and State Acts 2004, prohibiting people from suing firms for their obesity. The underlying principle was that people had to accept personal responsibility for their actions.[105]

One interesting outcome of the *Pelman* case is the market reaction; that is, the response firms have made to the threat of litigation by introducing healthy food offerings such as salads at McDonald's.[106] More generally, Daughety and Reinganum (1995) show that when liability is shifted toward suppliers, with low risk levels firms prefer to invest in cost saving (and price reducing) innovation activities, while high risks lead to research to improve product safety and healthiness. These results are consistent with other studies,[107] showing that liability directed at firms increases the intensity of research and development to improve product safety and

---

[102] See e.g. Miceli (2004).   [103] Adams (2005).
[104] Mello et al. (2003).   [105] Oliver (2006).
[106] According to Mello et al. (2003) this is the 'classical function of tort law as a deterrent of harmful behavior'.
[107] See e.g. Viscusi and Moore (1993).

healthiness, but this effect becomes negative above a certain level of liability as firms prefer to withdraw risky products from the market.

To summarize, the economic analysis of liability and obesity is limited and has focused on theory. Empirical economic research is needed to understand better what evidence exists on the desirability of liability rules.

Policy Evidence for Market Intervention Measures

From our perspective, public intervention that changes the external factors which drive consumer choice—relative prices—is more effective than information measures at changing consumer behavior and impacting on public health. Recent research suggests that combinations of fat tax and thin subsidy may have significant beneficial consequences for diets, particularly those of disadvantaged groups. Furthermore, a judicious fiscally neutral intervention need not impose a fiscal burden on the poor. From an economics perspective, an important argument for the fat tax is that it internalizes the externalities associated with obesity (medical costs and productivity losses; see Chapter 3). The fat tax does this by making people pay the true social cost of the foods they eat.

The measures we have discussed in this section are new and have not been evaluated for ex post effectiveness. As for information measures, we emphasize that interventions can have unintended side-effects, though these are not always negative. For example, a tax on unhealthy foods may lead firms to innovate to improve the health attributes of their products; and the threat of legal liability may encourage fast food chains to supply healthier alternatives to junk foods.

Although there is little hard quantitative evidence, most work suggests that controlling access of children to unhealthy food in schools is effective.

We reiterate the observation in the information section that obese people may respond differently from normal-weight people to economic incentives. We discussed how information about unhealthy eating provoked a dietary response only from the obese. Here we note that the children of obese parents were more likely to put on weight when junk foods are available in schools than the children of normal-weight parents. This distinction matters for evaluating policy interventions.

There are also cultural and traditional reasons why responses to policy measures of different socio-economic groups and different countries may vary. We reemphasize that policies are not necessarily transferable and ex ante analysis should avoid assuming a uniform response.

Conclusion

This chapter has discussed the details behind two groups of nutrition policy intervention tools: information measures and market intervention measures. Information measures can change knowledge and attitudes, but the evidence that they change behavior is weak. Few studies have attempted ex post evaluations of the costs and benefits of intervention. The limited evidence base suggests that nutrition labeling is uncontroversial, cheap, and necessary for those consumers who wish to make informed choices. But oversimplification in the form of front-of-pack color coding has the potential to misinform consumers and may provide inappropriate incentives to producers. Evidence is limited for the effectiveness of nutrition education, measures to restrict advertising of certain categories of food, and measures to promote the consumption of other categories through social marketing. These policies appear to influence knowledge and attitudes more than actual behavior. This does not necessarily mean that the policies should be scrapped. Consumers' welfare can be increased when information measures help them to make informed choices, even though they may not choose to eat more healthily.

Economic evaluation needs to be clear what it is trying to achieve: improved welfare through informed choice or reduced obesity through healthier eating. If the goal of policy intervention is to reduce externalities—the medical and productivity costs imposed by obese people on others—market intervention measures are more direct and more appropriate. Recent research suggests that well-thought-out combinations of fat taxes and thin subsidies may induce desirable changes in consumption while avoiding imposing an unfair burden on the poor. These measures deserve further consideration.

Disentangling the effectiveness of any particular tool remains a challenge, particularly because they are rarely introduced in isolation. Rather, they come within a package of measures, introduced simultaneously, preventing the opportunity to conduct the type of natural experiment that would enable us to measure policy effectiveness. For example, the famous North Karelia Project in Finland in 1972 was a 'comprehensive community-based program to control heart disease through life-style and risk factor changes'.[108] Less smoking and more exercise were emphasized along with better diet. Finnish heart disease mortality rates have fallen dramatically, but they began as the worst in Europe and remain worse than average. Have they improved because of less smoking, more exercise, better diets, or all three or none of the above? Perhaps the lower mortality rates were in part due to improvements in health care and medical technology. We know that the health improvements have not come through reduced obesity because since 1972 the Finns have become more obese. The final outcome of the public health intervention has been mediated by market forces, by medical progress, and by consumer choices, and a rigorous evaluation is needed to take into account these factors.

Although evidence on obesity policy is far from exhaustive, it seems to point in one direction. Information measures matter for informed consent and they may be effective in the case of information problems, but behavior does not always change, and more information does not translate into better health for the average person. Behavior is more likely to change in response to market measures, especially relative price changes achieved through a combination of fat taxes and thin subsidies, which can alter the allocation of consumption between unhealthy and healthy foods.

References

Adams, R. (2005), 'Fast Food, Obesity, and Tort Reform: An Examination of Industry Responsibility for Public Health', *Business and Society Review*, 110/3: 297–320.

Alderman, J., J. A. Smith, E. J. Fried, and R. A. Daynard (2007), 'Application of Law to the Childhood Obesity Epidemic', *Journal of Law, Medicine and Ethics*, 35/1: 90–112.

Alston, J. M. (2007), *Benefits and Beneficiaries from U.S. Farm Subsidies*, The 2007 Farm Bill & Beyond: Working Papers for the American Enterprise Institute for Public Policy Research.

——D. A. Sumner, and S. A. Vosti (2006), 'Are Agricultural Policies Making Us Fat? Likely Links between Agricultural Policies and Human Nutrition and Obesity, and their Policy Implications', *Review of Agricultural Economics*, 28/3: 313–22.

American Dietetic Association (2002), 'Position of the American Dietetic Association: Food and Nutrition Misinformation', *Journal of the American Dietetic Association*, 102/2: 260–6.

---

[108] Finnish National Public Health Institute, <http://www.ktl.fi>.

Anderson, P. M., and K. F. Butcher (2004), *Reading, Writing, and Raisinets: Are School Finances Contributing to Children's Obesity?*, Federal Reserve Bank of Chicago Working Paper 2004–16.

Armstrong, G. M. (1984), 'An Evaluation of the Children's Advertising Review Unit', *Journal of Public Policy and Marketing*, 3: 38–55.

——and M. Brucks (1988), 'Dealing with Children's Advertising: Public-Policy Issues and Alternatives', *Journal of Public Policy and Marketing*, 7: 98–113.

Ashton, D. (2004), 'Food Advertising and Childhood Obesity', *Journal of the Royal Society of Medicine*, 97/2: 51–2.

Balasubramanian, S. K., and C. Cole (2002), 'Consumers' Search and Use of Nutrition Information: The Challenge and Promise of the Nutrition Labeling and Education Act', *Journal of Marketing*, 66/3: 112–27.

Block, L. G., and L. A. Peracchio (2006), 'The Calcium Quandary: How Consumers Use Nutrition Labels', *Journal of Public Policy and Marketing*, 25/2: 188–96.

Bruce, A. (2000), 'Strategies to Prevent the Metabolic Syndrome at the Population Level: Role of Authorities and Non-Governmental Bodies', *British Journal of Nutrition*, 83: S181–S186.

Burton, S., E. H. Creyer, J. Kees, and K. Huggins (2006), 'Attacking the Obesity Epidemic: The Potential Health Benefits of Providing Nutrition Information in Restaurants', *American Journal of Public Health*, 96/9: 1669–75.

Bussell, G. (2005), 'Nutritional Profiling vs Guideline: Daily Amounts as a Means of Helping Consumers Make Appropriate Food Choices', *Nutrition and Food Science*, 35/5: 337–43.

Calfee, J. E. (2002), 'Public Policy Issues in Direct-to-Consumer Advertising of Prescription Drugs', *Journal of Public Policy and Marketing*, 21/2: 174–93.

Cash, S. B., D. L. Sunding, and D. Zilberman (2005), 'Fat Taxes and Thin Subsidies: Prices, Diet, and Health Outcomes', *Food Economics: Acta Agriculturae Scandinavica*, sect. C, 2/3–4: 167–74.

Cawley, J. (2006), 'Markets and Childhood Obesity Policy', *Future of Children*, 16/1: 69–88.

Chen, Z., S. T. Yen, and D. B. Eastwood (2005), 'Effects of Food Stamp Participation on Body Weight and Obesity', *American Journal of Agricultural Economics*, 87/5: 1167.

Chouinard, H. H., D. E. Davis, J. T. LaFrance, and J. M. Perloff (2007), 'Fat Taxes: Big Money for Small Change', *Forum for Health Economics and Policy*, 10/2, art. 2, <http://www.bepress.com/fhep/10/2/2>.

Clark, J. S., and J. W. Levedhal (2006), 'Will Fat Taxes Cause Americans to Become Fatter? Some Evidence from US Meats', Paper presented at the International Association of Agricultural Economists' Conference, Gold Coast, Australia, 12–18 Aug. 2006.

Collins, A., and M. McCarthy (2005), 'Top Shelf Foods and Drinks: Female Adolescents' Eating Motives, Constraints and Behaviors during the School Day', *Acta Agriculturae Scandinavica*, sect. C: *Economy*, 2/3–4: 205–13.

Coon, K. A., and K. L. Tucker (2002), 'Television and Children's Consumption Patterns: A Review of the Literature', *Minerva Pediatrica*, 54/5: 423–36.

Cresif (2004), 'Distribution de fruits dans les écoles maternelles et les collèges en réseau d'éducation prioritaire', Cresif Rapport d'exécution, Sept. 2004, <http://www.sante.gouv.fr/htm/pointsur/nutrition/rapport_final_dgs_fruits4.pdf>.

Dallongeville, J., N. Marecaux, D. Cottel, A. Bingham, and P. Amouyel (2001), 'Association between Nutrition Knowledge and Nutritional Intake in Middle-Aged Men from Northern France', *Public Health Nutrition*, 4/1: 27–33.

Dalmeny, K., E. Hanna, and T. Lobstein (2004), 'Broadcasting Bad Health: Why Food Marketing to Children Needs to Be Controlled', *Journal of the HEIA*, 11/1–2: 10–46.

Daughety, A. F., and J. F. Reinganum (1995), 'Product Safety: Liability, R & D, and Signaling', *American Economic Review*, 85/5: 1187–1206.

Duecy, E. (2006), 'Chain QSR Market Share Growing in Big European Markets', *Nation's Restaurant News*, 40/37: 16–17.

Dunkelberger, E., and S. E. Taylor (1993), 'The NLEA, Health Claims, and the 1st Amendment', *Food and Drug Law Journal*, 48/4: 631–64.

Finkelstein, E. A., S. French, J. N. Variyam, and P. S. Haines (2004), 'Pros and Cons of Proposed Interventions to Promote Healthy Eating', *American Journal of Preventive Medicine*, 27/3: 163–71.

Foster, W., and R. E. Just (1989), 'Measuring Welfare Effects of Product Contamination with Consumer Uncertainty', *Journal of Environmental Economics and Management*, 17/3: 266–83.

Fox, J., D. Hayes, and J. Shogren (2002), 'Consumer Preferences for Food Irradiation: How Favorable and Unfavorable Descriptions Affect Preferences for Irradiated Pork in Experimental Auctions', *Journal of Risk and Uncertainty*, 24: 75–95.

French, S. A. (2005), 'Population Approaches to Promote Healthful Eating Behaviors', in D. Crawford and R. W. Jeffery (eds), *Obesity Prevention and Public Health* (Oxford: Oxford University Press).

——M. Story, J. A. Fulkerson, and A. F. Gerlach (2003), 'Food Environment in Secondary Schools: À la Carte, Vending Machines, and Food Policies and Practices', *American Journal of Public Health*, 93/7: 1161–7.

Garretson, J. A., and S. Burton (2000), 'Effects of Nutrition Facts, Panel Values, Nutrition Claims, and Health Claims on Consumer Attitudes, Perceptions of Disease-Related Risks, and Trust', *Journal of Public Policy and Marketing*, 19/2: 213–27.

Goel, R. K., and M. A. Nelson (2006), 'The Effectiveness of Anti-Smoking Legislation: A Review', *Journal of Economic Surveys*, 20/3: 325–55.

Golan, E., F. Kuchler, L. Mitchell, C. Greene, and A. Jessup (2001), 'Economics of Food Labeling', *Journal of Consumer Policy*, 24/2: 117–84.

Gordon, R., L. McDermott, M. Stead, and K. Angus (2006), 'The Effectiveness of Social Marketing Interventions for Health Improvement: What's the Evidence?', *Public Health*, 120/12: 1133–9.

Grunert, K. G., and J. M. Wills (2007), 'A Review of European Research on Consumer Response to Nutrition Information on Food Labels', *Journal of Public Health*, 15/5: 385–99.

Halpern, D., C. Bates, G. Beales, and A. Heathfield (2004), *Personal Responsibility and Changing Behavior: The State of Knowledge and its Implications for Public Policy* (London: Cabinet Office, Prime Minister's Strategy Unit).

Hartmann, M., A. K. Lensch, J. Simons, and S. Thrams (2005), 'Nutrition and Health Claims: Information or Deception', Paper presented at the 97th EAAE Seminar, Reading, 21–2 Apr.

Hastings, G., M. Stead, L. McDermott, A. Forsyth, A. M. MacKintosh, M. Rayner, C. Godfrey, M. Caraher, and K. Angus (2003), *Review of Research on the Effects of Food Promotion to Children*, Report prepared for the Food Standard Agency (Strathclyde: University of Strathclyde, Centre for Social Marketing).

Hawkes, C. (2004), *Marketing Food to Children: The Global Regulatory Environment* (Geneva: World Health Organization).

Hofferth, S. L., and S. Curtin (2005), 'Poverty, Food Programs, and Childhood Obesity', *Journal of Policy Analysis and Management*, 24/4: 703–26.

Ippolito, P. M., and J. K. Pappalardo (2002), 'Advertising Nutrition and Health: Evidence from Food Advertising', Bureau of Economics Staff Report, Federal Trade Commission, Washington, DC, 20580, Sept. 2002.

Jacobson, M. F., and K. D. Brownell (2000), 'Small Taxes on Soft Drinks and Snack Foods to Promote Health', *American Journal of Public Health*, 90/6: 854–7.

Jargon, J. (2006), 'The King Is Lurking', *Crain's Chicago Business*, 29/39: 3–10.

Kan, K., and W. D. Tsai (2004), 'Obesity and Risk Knowledge', *Journal of Health Economics*, 23/5: 907–34.

Kaushal, N. (2007), 'Do Food Stamps Cause Obesity? Evidence from Immigrant Experience', *Journal of Health Economics*, 26/5: 968–91.

Kral, T. V. E., L. S. Roe, and B. J. Rolls (2002), 'Does Nutrition Information about the Energy Density of Meals Affect Food Intake in Normal-Weight Women?', *Appetite*, 39/2: 137–45.

Krebs, J. (2004), 'What's on the Label?', *Science*, 306/5699: 1101.

Kuchler, F., E. Golan, J. N. Variyam, and S. R. Crutchfield (2005a), 'Obesity Policy and the Law of Unintended Consequences', *Amber Waves*, 3/3: 26–33.

——A. Tegene, and J. M. Harris (2005b), 'Taxing Snack Foods: Manipulating Diet Quality or Financing Information Programs?', *Review of Agricultural Economics*, 27/1: 4–20.

Lafontaine, F. (1995), *Pricing Decisions in Franchised Chains: A Look at the Restaurant and Fast-Food Industry*, NBER Working Papers 5247 (Cambridge, Mass.: National Bureau of Economic Research).

Larsson, I., L. Lissner, and L. Wilhelmsen (1999), 'The "Green Keyhole" Revisited: Nutritional Knowledge May Influence Food Selection', *European Journal of Clinical Nutrition*, 53/10: 776–80.

Leather, S. (1996), 'The CAP Regime for Fruit and Vegetables', in M. Whitehead and P. Nordgren (eds), *Health Impact Assessment of the EU Common Agricultural Policy* (Stockholm: Swedish National Institute of Public Health).

Leicester, A., and F. Windmeijer (2004), *The 'Fat Tax': Economic Incentives to Reduce Obesity*, IFS Briefing Notes BN49.

Lobstein, T. (2002), 'Food Policies: A Threat to Health?', *Proceedings of the Nutrition Society*, 61/4: 579–85.

Marshall, T. (2000), 'Exploring a Fiscal Food Policy: The Case of Diet and Ischaemic Heart Disease', *British Medical Journal*, 320/7230: 301–4.

Mazzocchi, M., and W. B. Traill (2005), 'Nutrition, Health and Economic Policies in Europe', *Food Economics: Acta Agriculturae Scandinavica*, sect. C, 2/3: 138–49.

Mello, M. M., E. B. Rimm, and D. M. Studdert (2003), 'The McLawsuit: The Fast-Food Industry and Legal Accountability for Obesity', *Health Affairs*, 22/6: 207–16.

Miceli, T. J. (2004), *The Economic Approach to Law* (Stanford, Calif.: Stanford University Press).

Miller, D. L., V. H. Castellanos, D. J. Shide, J. C. Peters, and B. J. Rolls (1998), 'Effect of Fat-Free Potato Chips with and without Nutrition Labels on Fat and Energy Intakes', *American Journal of Clinical Nutrition*, 68/2: 282–90.

Miller, J. C., and K. H. Coble (2007), 'Cheap Food Policy: Fact or Rhetoric?', *Food Policy*, 32/1: 98–111.

Mytton, O., A. Gray, M. Rayner, and H. Rutter (2007), 'Could Targeted Food Taxes Improve Health?', *Journal of Epidemiology and Community Health*, 61/8: 689–94.

NARC (2004), *White Paper: Guidance for Food Advertising Self-Regulation* (New York: National Advertising Review Council).

Nelson, J. P. (2003a), 'Youth Smoking Prevalence in Developing Countries: Effect of Advertising Bans', *Applied Economics Letters*, 10/13: 805–11.

——(2003b), 'Cigarette Demand, Structural Change, and Advertising Bans: International Evidence, 1970–1995', *Contributions to Economic Analysis and Policy*, 2/1: a10.

Nestle, M. (2000), 'Changing the Diet of a Nation: Population/Regulatory Strategies for a Developed Economy', *Asia Pacific Journal of Clinical Nutrition*, 9: S33–S40.

Oliver, J. E. (2006), *Fat Politics: The Real Story behind America's Obesity Epidemic* (New York: Oxford University Press).

Pappalardo, J. K. (1996), 'Evaluating the NLEA: Where's the Beef?', *Journal of Public Policy and Marketing*, 15/1: 153–6.

——and D. J. Ringold (2000), 'Regulating Commercial Speech in a Dynamic Environment: Forty Years of Margarine and Oil Advertising before the NLEA', *Journal of Public Policy and Marketing*, 19/1: 74–92.

Petruccelli, P. J. (1996), 'Consumer and Marketing Implications of Information Provision: The Case of the Nutrition Labeling and Education Act of 1990', *Journal of Public Policy and Marketing*, 15/1: 150–3.

Petty, R. D. (1997), 'Advertising Law in the United States and European Union', *Journal of Public Policy and Marketing*, 16/1: 2–13.

Pollard, C. M., M. R. Miller, A. M. Daly, K. E. Crouchley, K. J. Donoghue, A. J. Lang, and C. W. Binns (2007), 'Increasing Fruit and Vegetable Consumption: Success of the Western Australian Go for 2 & 5 Campaign', *Public Health Nutrition*, 11/03: 314–20.

Prattala, R. (2003), 'Dietary Changes in Finland: Success Stories and Future Challenges', *Appetite*, 41/3: 245–9.

Prevention Institute (2002), 'Restricting Television Advertising to Children', Nutrition Policy Profile, May 2002, <http://www.preventioninstitute.org/CHI_food_advertising.html>.

Puska, P. (2002), 'Successful Prevention of Non-Communicable Diseases: 25 Year Experiences with North Karelia Project in Finland', *Public Health Medicine*, 4/1: 5–7.

Rindfleisch, A., and D. X. Crockett (1999), 'Cigarette Smoking and Perceived Risk: A Multidimensional Investigation', *Journal of Public Policy and Marketing*, 18/2: 159–71.

Ritson, C. (1991), 'The CAP and the Consumer', in C. Ritson and A. Harvey (eds), *The Common Agricultural Policy and the World Economy* (Wallingford: CAB Publishing).

—— (1998), 'Agenda 2000', *Nutrition and Food Science*, 98/4: 198–201.

Roe, B., A. S. Levy, and B. M. Derby (1999), 'The Impact of Health Claims on Consumer Search and Product Evaluation Outcomes: Results from FDA Experimental Data', *Journal of Public Policy and Marketing*, 18/1: 89–105.

Roos, G., M. Lean, and A. Anderson (2002), 'Dietary Interventions in Finland, Norway and Sweden: Nutrition Policies and Strategies', *Journal of Human Nutrition and Dietetics*, 15/2: 99–110.

Saffer, H., and F. Chaloupka (2000), 'The Effect of Tobacco Advertising Bans on Tobacco Consumption', *Journal of Health Economics*, 19/6: 1117–37.

Schafer-Elinder, L. (2003), *Public Health Aspects of the EU Common Agricultural Policy* (Stockholm: Swedish National Institute of Public Health).

—— (2004), 'The EU Common Agricultural Policy from a Public Health Perspective', *Eurohealth*, 10/1: 13–16.

Seiders, K., and R. D. Petty (2004), 'Obesity and the Role of Food Marketing: A Policy Analysis of Issues and Remedies', *Journal of Public Policy and Marketing*, 23/2: 153–69.

Sheehan, K. B. (2003), 'Balancing Acts: An Analysis of Food and Drug Administration Letters about Direct-to-Consumer Advertising Violations', *Journal of Public Policy and Marketing*, 22/2: 159–69.

Silverglade, B. A. (1991), 'Public-Policy Issues in Health Claims for Foods: Comment', *Journal of Public Policy and Marketing*, 10/1: 54–62.

—— (1996), 'The Nutrition Labeling and Education Act: Progress to Date and Challenges for the Future', *Journal of Public Policy and Marketing*, 15/1: 148–50.

Skinner, T., H. Miller, and C. Bryant (2005), 'The Literature on the Economic Causes of and Policy Responses to Obesity', *Food Economics: Acta Agriculturae Scandinavica*, sect. C, 2/3–4: 128–37.

Smed, S., J. D. Jensen, and S. Denver (2007), 'Socio-economic Characteristics and the Effect of Taxation as a Health Policy Instrument', *Food Policy*, 32/5–6: 624–39.

Stead, M., G. Hastings, and L. McDermott (2007), 'The Meaning, Effectiveness and Future of Social Marketing', *Obesity Reviews*, 8: 189–93.

Story, M., and S. French (2004), 'Food Advertising and Marketing Directed at Children and Adolescents in the US', *International Journal of Behavioral Nutrition and Physical Activity*, 1/1: 3–17.

—— K. M. Kaphingst, and S. French (2006), 'The Role of Schools in Obesity Prevention', *Future of Children*, 16/1: 109–42.

Stubenitsky, K., J. I. Aaron, S. L. Catt, and D. J. Mela (2000), 'The Influence of Recipe Modification and Nutritional Information on Restaurant Food Acceptance and Macronutrient Intakes', *Public Health Nutrition*, 3/02: 201–9.

Swinburn, B. A., I. Caterson, J. C. Seidell, and W. P. T. James (2004), 'Diet, Nutrition and the Prevention of Excess Weight Gain and Obesity', *Public Health Nutrition*, 7/1a: 123–46.

Teisl, M. F., N. E. Bockstael, and A. Levy (2001), 'Measuring the Welfare Effects of Nutrition Information', *American Journal of Agricultural Economics*, 83/1: 133–49.

Thirtle, C. G., D. E. Schimmelpfennig, and R. F. Townsend (2002), 'Induced Innovation in United States Agriculture, 1880–1990: Time Series Tests and an Error Correction Model', *American Journal of Agricultural Economics*, 84/3: 598–614.

Tillotson, J. E. (2004), 'America's Obesity: Conflicting Public Policies, Industrial Economic Development, and Unintended Human Consequences', *Annual Review of Nutrition*, 24: 617–43.

Variyam, J. N. (2004), *Nutrition Labeling in the Food-away-from-Home Sector: An Economic Assessment*, USDA-ERS Economic Research Report 4.

—— and J. Cawley (2006), *Nutrition Labels and Obesity*, NBER Working Papers 11956 (Cambridge, Mass.: National Bureau of Economic Research).

Ver Ploeg, M., L. Mancino, B. H. Lin, and C. Y. Wang (2007), 'The Vanishing Weight Gap: Trends in Obesity among Adult Food Stamp Participants (US) (1976–2002)', *Economics and Human Biology*, 5/1: 20–36.

Viner, R. M., and T. J. Cole (2005), 'Television Viewing in Early Childhood Predicts Adult Body Mass Index', *Journal of Pediatrics*, 147/4: 429–35.

Viscusi, W. K., and M. J. Moore (1993), 'Product Liability, Research-and-Development, and Innovation', *Journal of Political Economy*, 101/1: 161–84.

von Haartman, F. (1996), 'The CAP Regime for Dairy Products', in M. Whitehead and P. Nordgren (eds), *Health Impact Assessment of the EU Common Agricultural Policy* (Stockholm: Swedish National Institute of Public Health).

Whitmore Schanzenbach, D. (2005), *Do School Lunches Contribute to Childhood Obesity?*, Harris School Working Papers, ser. 5, 13 (Chicago: University of Chicago, Harris School of Public Policy).

Wootan, M. G., and M. Osborn (2006), 'Availability of Nutrition Information from Chain Restaurants in the United States', *American Journal of Preventive Medicine*, 30/3: 266–8.

Zywicki, T. J., D. Holt, and M. K. Ohlhausen (2004), 'Obesity and Advertising Policy', *George Mason Law Review*, 12/4: 979–1011.

5

Conclusion

The World Health Organization predicts that by 2015 nearly 2.3 billion adults (aged 15+) will be overweight and over 700 million will be obese, increases of almost 50% on current estimates of about 1.6 billion overweight and 400 million obese adults. The general fear is that this rapid rise of overweight and obese people will create even greater demand for scarce medical services and generate even more extra costs on society as a whole—unless people choose to change their behavior themselves or through government or third party policy intervention. Understanding the potential consequences of obesity and evaluating alternative solutions requires a coherent framework that can balance options with costs of achieving them. Economics provides such a framework: a useful tool to organize one's thinking about the trade-offs involved in allowing personal choices given social goals.

We have argued that the obesity challenge must account for basic principles of economic behavior to avoid wasting valuable resources. We examine why economics matters more to health and obesity than people think, and what this implies for the ongoing debate over how to implement policies to improve health around the globe. We recognize that economics should not be confused with the morality of setting health standards. That said, not everyone agrees with the moral argument of 'better health regardless of the cost', the dominant view in the health debate. Election data, government budget allocations, and agency behavior demonstrate that current moral outrage falls short of generating the political will necessary to impose strict regulations and rules that would outlaw unhealthy diets or impose mandatory exercise regimes. And although people support the goal of better human health, people would not choose to impose strict regulations if doing so would divert resources from other goals such as climate protection, education, and a decent standard of living. In reality, obesity policy is as much a question of social choice as of biology.

We conclude *Fat Economics* with seven points based on our understanding of the economics of obesity.

1. *Obesity poses a modern day challenge to understanding human health and welfare.* The 'obesity epidemic' in the developed world is 20 years old. But since its emergence as a 'major public health concern', deaths from obesity-related diseases such as heart disease, stroke, and diabetes have fallen sharply. These seemingly contradictory data lead one to conclude that obesity has become less dangerous and normal people need to make fewer sacrifices to avoid gaining weight; excess weight is a rational outcome of people's balancing their individual risks and benefits.

2. *Obesity seems to be due to technological change.* Technology has lowered the cost of food, and the cheapest food can be the least healthy food. Food has become cheaper, especially processed and fast foods; and the time cost of food consumption has fallen as mass preparation has taken over from individual preparation. People have responded to these incentives by consuming more processed and fast foods and snack foods. The average person's lifestyle has also become less energy-demanding, both at work and in leisure time, owing to the reduction of manual work and the growing availability of transport.

3. *Obesity and its related health problems are as much an economics issue as they are a biological problem.* Economists concur that policy should be evidence-based; but they also argue that economics should play a more central role, not just be called on to calculate cost-effectiveness. People respond to economic incentives. Consumer behavior responds in a predictable way to changes in relative prices, incomes, or the time cost of food preparation. Producers respond in a rational, but sometimes less predictable, way, reformulating products to improve labels, investing in new technologies. Economics defines the potential social costs and benefits from an intervention, assesses consumers' and producers' likely response to the incentives provided by legislation, and identifies data and methods needed for subsequent ex post evaluation of the intervention. In addition, common myths about obesity deserve a deeper analysis based on economic reasoning. It is not the case that agricultural policies have favored rising obesity rates. If any effect exists, it may even be positive. Recall that retail prices partially reflect farm prices. Supported farm prices have made food more expensive and the Common Agricultural Policy has altered relative prices in a positive way.

4. *Obesity policy needs economics for both risk assessment and risk management.* Establishing health goals is accomplished by assessing the likelihood of death and illness. Here economics plays a role in determining health states because human choices and adaptation to economic parameters affect the odds of survival and disease. The key variables in economic and health systems are jointly determined; neither health quality nor economics is autonomous. The feedback loop between economic choices and health needs to be better accounted for in obesity policy. In considering the future trajectory of obesity and health, policymakers must account for economic parameters. This view challenges the traditional risk assessment–management bifurcation in which risk is first quantified by the natural or life sciences and then recovery strategies are evaluated by economists. At the onset, proper risk assessment should incorporate parameters from both the biological and the economic systems. There is the question of whether the benefits of gathering economic information to improve the implementation of obesity policy exceed the costs of data collection and the resulting delays in decision making. Evidence from parallel efforts with other public policy issues suggests that they do: the net benefits from economic information are positive. When economics enters the picture, the target is not health any more, it is the wider concept of welfare. This implies that different people may have different routes to happiness: fair obesity policies need to take this into account, together with an accurate evaluation of the distribution of costs and benefits.

5. *Obesity warrants government intervention in the marketplace if obese people impose costs on the rest of society. In other cases, market failure must be shown.* In determining whether the obesity epidemic merits a government response one must consider whether it is a result of market failure. Market failure can result from consumers having imperfect information about diet and health or through externalities—obese people imposing costs on the rest of society. Such external costs of obesity justify public intervention if the non-obese support the costs generated by obese people. This is likely to happen in public health care systems. But government intervention is not necessarily justified when consumer choices are free and fully informed. This case of informed consent seems to exist in most developed countries, while information biases may exist. Specific cases exist which require government intervention, but these should not be generalized to the national or worldwide level. Children are one case since they lack self-control and are more easily influenced by marketing actions. In addition, some markets can be less competitive than others; for

example, there is strong concentration in the fast food industry, which suggests that information on health and food is skewed.

6. *Obesity cannot be changed by information policy alone. The average person becomes more knowledgeable but he or she does not necessarily change his or her behavior.* Improved information is essential for informed choice, but may not promote healthier eating. It may still improve welfare. Information measures by themselves are rarely effective. Public information measures are widely employed but they only affect the demand side; if supply does not react, the final outcome might be a price increase. Furthermore, public information measures act on attitudes and intentions, but the evidence on behavioral change is weak. Actual empirical analysis confirms that information interventions are relatively ineffective at combating obesity. Most interesting things happen in the right-hand tail of the BMI distribution in terms of response to economic incentives and to information measures. On reflection, this is not surprising. For example, why should a normal-weight person change his or her diet in response to a message that obesity is bad for health?

7. *Obesity can be addressed by a policy combination of fat taxes and thin subsidies.* Given that unhealthy eating imposes externalities (medical costs, productivity) the true social cost of unhealthy diets is not reflected in the market price. Market measures, when justified by market failure, are more effective because they redress imbalances between private and social costs. But there may be distributional implications to account for when taxes are regressive. A combination of taxes on unhealthy foods and subsidies on healthy foods might be the solution. Judiciously chosen, the financial burden need not fall disproportionately on the poor—who would benefit most in health outcomes from these measures. That said, there is still concern that the poor will pay disproportionately to solve the problem.

Just as policymakers cannot ignore the laws of nature, neither can they ignore the laws of human nature when thinking about obesity and health policy. Economic behavior matters for obesity, given that the choices on what we eat and how we exercise depend on the relative prices of food and leisure. Effective policy at all levels requires that we adjust our perspectives to integrate better both human actions and their reactions to health risk into the mix of viewpoints guiding obesity policy.

Glossary

availability (of food, energy, calories . . .) Availability is often used as a proxy for consumption and is obtained as the difference between production and all other uses before food reaches the retail level (net exports, feed, production and processing waste, industrial usage, stock change, etc.). This is the method used by FAO in their Supply Utilization Accounts and Food Balance Sheets to estimate food and calorie consumption. Example: *milk consumption in Italy = (production in Italy + imports to Italy + beginning stocks) – (exports from Italy + waste + other non-food uses + ending stocks)*. Food availability generally overestimates consumption, because it ignores household waste, which can be around 20% for perishable foods like milk or fruit.

basal metabolic rate (BMR) Roughly, it is the minimum amount of energy (calories) needed to survive while inactive. Typically, it is measured on individuals woken up after 8 hours of sleep and 12 hours of fasting (to ensure no digestion), with the subject resting in a reclining position. The BMR has been found to be influenced by age (negatively), height (positively), weight (positively), with differences between men and women.

body mass index (BMI) The ratio between the weight of an individual in kilograms and his/her squared height in meters. Individuals are classified as underweight when their BMI is below 18.5, overweight when it is between 25 and 30, and obese when it is above 30.

bounded rationality In economics, bounded rationality relaxes the common assumption that individuals can make perfectly rational decisions to maximize their satisfaction (utility). In practice, perfect rationality is prevented by difficulties in complex optimizing behavior (e.g. choosing among 20 types of yoghurt compared to choosing between two types), and by the cost and effort needed to gather and process information. Thus, economic agents tend to simplify their decisions by using *heuristics. See Chapter 2.

brand In marketing, a brand is the mix of psychological and experiential aspects associated with a company or product (usually through symbols like names, logos, etc.). The expression 'brand image' usually refers to the psychological aspects.

brand share   *See* market (brand) share.

brand switching   In marketing, brand switching refers to the consumer decision to buy a different brand from the one usually purchased.

budget constraint   In *consumer theory, the budget constraint defines the bundle of goods and services that a consumer can buy given his/her income and the market prices. See Chapter 2.

childhood obesity   The definition of childhood obesity differs from that of adult obesity because the BMI in childhood changes substantially with age. Hence, age- and sex-specific cut-off points to define childhood obesity (overweight) from 2 to 18 years are often used instead of BMI. See Chapter 1.

Common Agricultural Policy (CAP)   The CAP is a policy system implemented in the European Union which supports farmers through direct farm income subsidies and commodity-specific price support mechanisms.

consumer theory   A theory of microeconomics to model consumer demand based on a set of rationality assumptions on the structure of consumer preferences (completeness, reflexivity, and transitivity). Rational preferences must also fulfill the axioms of non-satiation (larger bundles are preferred to smaller ones) and convexity (roughly that the additional satisfaction for consuming larger quantities is decreasing). With rational preferences and subject to a budget constraint, consumers make their choice in order to maximize their overall satisfaction (*utility). Theory-based demand models are used to explain consumption choices on the basis of changes in relative prices and real income. *See also* bounded rationality; Chapter 2.

contingent valuation (CV)   An economic technique to 'monetize' non-market goods, i.e. assign a monetary value to goods which are not marketed (e.g. clean air). With CV, monetization is based on stated-preferences surveys, where respondents express their *willingness-to-pay or *willingness-to-accept for these non-market resources.

control group   In scientific experimental settings, two groups are compared to test the influence of a given factor. The target or treatment group is subject to the factor, while the control group must have the same characteristics as the target group, except that it is not subject to the factor. By comparing the outcomes of the interest variable between the two groups, it becomes possible to elicit the influence of the factor. For example, one might compare the health outcomes of a target group of obese patients compared to a control group of non-obese patients, where individuals in the control group must be as similar as possible to those in the target group, except for their BMI, to avoid the influence of other confounding factors.

correlation   A statistical measure of the strength of association between two quantitative variables which varies between −1 (an increase in one variable exactly corresponds to a decrease in the other variable) and 1 (an increase in one variable exactly corresponds to an increase in the other variable), where a 0 correlation means that the two variables are unrelated.

cost–benefit analysis An economic procedure to evaluate the case for a project (e.g. a policy intervention) on the basis of the costs and benefits of the intervention, relative to the status quo. Costs and benefits include direct monetary effects, non-monetary effects (which may be quantified through techniques like *contingent valuation), and opportunity costs (the cost of resources in their best alternative use). *See also* Chapter 3.

cost-effectiveness analysis An economic procedure which relates the costs of alternative interventions which achieve the same outcome (e.g. the cost per life saved). A special case is *cost–utility analysis. *See also* Chapter 3.

cost-of-ignorance The monetary-equivalent cost suffered by economic agents when they take decisions based on wrong information.

cost-of-illness A procedure to quantify the direct costs associated with a given health condition, based on the costs associated with medical diagnosis, treatment, and follow-up care, like physicians' visits, hospitalization, and pharmaceuticals. Indirect costs such as forgone wages and lost productivity may also be accounted for. *See also* Chapter 3.

cost–utility analysis A special case of *cost-effectiveness analysis, where the outcomes are measured in terms of *quality adjusted life years or *disability adjusted life years. *See also* Chapter 3.

counterfactual In policy evaluation studies, the counterfactual of an intervention is the outcome that would have been observed without the intervention. *See also* Chapter 3.

difference-in-difference A non-experimental method to evaluate the impact of a policy intervention. It compares the outcome of the intervention in a treatment and *control group, not in terms of absolute levels, but in terms of the differences between the level of the outcome before and after the intervention in both groups. The procedure thus controls for dynamics which are not influenced by the intervention. *See also* Chapter 3.

disability adjusted life years (DALYs) A measure of the burden of disease which combines years of life lost and years lived with disability. One DALY corresponds to one year of healthy life lost. *See also* quality adjusted life years; Chapter 2.

distribution *See* frequency distribution.

disutility A negative impact on *utility.

economic growth The change in a country's wealth, usually measured as percentage change in real gross domestic product.

economies of scale These are the reduction in the cost per unit of output associated with an expansion of output. For example, the cost per hamburger might be $1 for a firm producing 1,000 hamburgers per day compared to $0.5 for a firm producing 100,000 hamburgers per day, thanks to size-associated savings in inputs like labor, technology, etc.

elasticity *See* price elasticity; income elasticity.

endogeneity In economics, a variable within a model is said to be endogenous when its change comes from inside the model. The model can be thus exploited to explain changes in endogenous variables. For example, in a supply–demand model, prices are endogenous as they change as a function of changes in demand and supply. Price levels and changes can be thus explained by a supply–demand model. *See also* exogeneity.

ex ante policy evaluation A policy evaluation procedure aimed at quantifying the impact of an intervention before it takes place. *See also* ex post policy evaluation; Chapter 3.

exogeneity In economics, a variable within a model is exogenous when its change does not come from inside the model, but is determined outside the model. Exogenous variables determine changes in endogenous variables (*see* endogeneity), but endogenous variables do not determine changes in exogenous variables. For example, the tax rate is exogenous in a demand model, as the tax rate influences demand, but (generally) demand does not influence the tax rate.

expected utility When an economic decision has uncertain outcomes, expected utility measures the average utility, measured as the weighted average of the utility of all possible outcomes, using the probability of each outcome as the weights.

ex post policy evaluation A policy evaluation procedure aimed at quantifying the impact of an intervention after the intervention has been completed. *See also* ex ante policy evaluation; Chapter 3.

externality An economic side-effect (which can be either positive or negative) generated by an economic activity but not reflected by prices.

farm support An intervention aimed at supporting farm income, for example by artificially maintaining prices at a higher level than the market price (price support) or through direct subsidies to income.

fat tax A tax on energy-dense or nutrient-poor food.

Food Stamp Program A US federal program to subsidize food consumption of low- and no-income people.

frequency distribution   The complete set of values of a given variable, possibly grouped into classes, together with the frequency they appear in a sample or population.

functional form   The shape of a function which expresses the relationship between two or more variables.

generic advertising   An advertising strategy not targeted at a specific brand, but promoting an entire category of a product (e.g. promoting apple consumption).

guideline daily amount (GDA)   The recommended daily intake of a nutrient considered healthy for an everyday diet.

habit formation   The process determining the persistence of consumption habits. Habit formation is observed when current consumption depends on past consumption.

health claims   Claims (on food labels, adverts, etc.) by food manufacturers about the positive health impact of consumption of their food. According to current regulations, they need to be substantiated by scientific research.

heuristic   Rule of thumb, based on readily accessible information, to take quick decisions. Economic agents use heuristics especially in situations requiring complex problem solving. *See also* bounded rationality.

household production function   An economic model which sees the household as a production and consumption unit which uses time as leisure or to generate income to purchase goods and services including leisure activities such as gym subscriptions to generate outputs, like health. Thus, consumer *utility depends on both direct pleasure from consumption and the effect of other outputs (e.g. adverse health effect from consumption). *See* Box 2.1; Chapter 2.

incidence (of a disease)   The proportion of new onsets of a disease with respect to the population potentially at risk over a given period of time (usually a year). It is a measure of the probability of developing a condition. *See also* prevalence.

income elasticity   In economics, responsiveness of consumption to changes in income, expressed as the percentage change in consumption generated by a 1% change in income.

income quartiles   A subdivision of a population (or sample) into four categories ordered according to income level, where each category includes 25% of the total population.

information asymmetry   In economics, a situation where economic agents participating in the market have different levels of information. For example, producers of a food have better information on the ingredients and production process than consumers.

intra-household allocation The process at the household level which determines purchasing decisions and the allocation of consumption among the members of the same household.

labor force participation The ratio of population which is in the workforce, intended as all those people who can work (employed, unemployed, and those looking for a job). For example, age- and gender-specific labor force participation rate (e.g. female participation rate) can be computed.

legal liability In law, the responsibility of an individual or a company to pay compensation for any damage incurred because of a tort for which the individual (company) is liable. See Chapter 4.

long-run (equilibrium) In economics, the time-span needed by the market to reach a stable equilibrium. There is no consensus about the length of this time-span.

market (brand) share The share of sales for a specific brand as a proportion of total sales in the same product category.

market (economic) equilibrium A steady state of the market resulting from the balance of economic forces.

market failure A market outcome where the allocation of goods is not economically efficient because of externalities, imperfect information, or market power. *See also* Chapter 2.

market power A departure from perfect competition, where some economic agents have the power to alter or control price. *See e.g.* monopoly; oligopoly.

monopoly A market with a single producer.

obese *See* body mass index.

oligopoly A departure from perfect competition, where the number of economic agents is small, so each can adopt strategic behavior by taking into account the likely response of other agents.

opportunity cost The value of the benefits one could have received by taking an alternative decision from the one being considered.

overweight *See* body mass index.

paternalism Policy that makes public decisions for economic agents with the intent of protecting them or improving their welfare at the expense of their freedom of action; for example, a policy forbidding alcohol or fatty foods to protect public health.

percentiles The cut-off values of a variable below which lies a given proportion of the population (or sample). For example, the 90th percentile of BMI is the value below which 90% of the observations fall.

perfect competition A market where no individual producer or consumer is able to influence prices. In microeconomic theory, perfect competition leads to an efficient market equilibrium. Perfect competition requires large numbers of producers and consumers, no barriers to entry, perfect information, substitutability of products, and independent decisions of economic agents. *See also* monopoly; oligopoly; market power.

physical activity (measurement of) Measurement of physical activity is usually based on four dimensions: (1) the frequency with which physical activity is undertaken (e.g. days per week); (2) duration per session (e.g. 30 minutes); (3) intensity based on self-perception or classified according to calorie consumption (e.g. light, moderate, vigorous); (4) domain of physical activity (e.g. leisure time, occupational, domestic). An adequate physical activity consists of 30 minutes of moderate walking at least 5 days per week.

preferences In economics, preferences or tastes reflect the possibility of rank ordering consumption choices, based on the satisfaction (*utility) they provide. Each consumer has his/her individual preference structure, which is reflected in the *utility function.

prevalence (of a disease) The proportion of existing cases of a given disease in the total population at a given time. It differs from *incidence, which records new cases in a given time period.

price elasticity This measures the responsiveness of consumption to price changes, as the percentage change in consumption induced by a 1% change in price. If the price being considered is the price of the good itself, it is called own-price elasticity. If the objective is to measure responsiveness to changes in the price of a substitute good, it is called cross-price elasticity.

private costs The costs actually borne by economic agents in their production and consumption activities. In well-functioning markets, private costs are equal to *social costs.

productivity (of labor, capital) The amount of output per labor (capital) unit.

proxy variable A variable which can act as an appropriate substitute for another variable which is not available. For example, urbanization may be used as a proxy for physical activity levels.

quality adjusted life years (QALYs) Similarly to *disability adjusted life years, QALYs are obtained to estimate the burden of disease by applying weights to years lived with a given condition, where the weights depend on the quality of life. The quality of life is assessed on the basis of survey, with various elicitation methods. *See also* Chapter 2.

rational addiction A form of addictive consumption which is consistent with the rationality assumption. Consumers are both backward- and forward-looking and take their decisions according to an optimal consumption plan which takes into consideration both present and future consumption. *See also* Chapter 2.

rational choice *See* consumer theory.

raw commodities Primary products that are not subject to industry processing.

real income The adjustment of current income for inflation. It is measured by dividing current income by the current price index with respect to a given base year. Real income is thus a measure of purchasing power relative to the base year.

real prices The adjustment of current prices for inflation. It is measured by dividing current prices by the current price index with respect to a given base year.

real rate of return (on investments) The ratio of money gained or lost on an investment relative to the amount of money invested, after adjusting for inflation.

regressive effect of taxation A tax is said to be regressive when it falls disproportionately on those with lower incomes. For example, a *fat tax might be regressive as the amount of unhealthy nutrients consumed decreases at higher-income level. *See also* Chapter 4.

relative prices Prices expressed as the ratio to other prices. For example, if the relative price of apples in terms of the price of oranges is 1.5, it means that apples cost 50% more than oranges.

risk analysis The assessment, management, and communication of risks.

risk assessment The first step of *risk analysis, which consists of the quantification (or qualitative evaluation) of potential risks.

risk aversion The inclination of an individual to take or avoid risk. Higher risk aversion means less inclination to take risks.

risk communication The third step of *risk analysis is the process of exchanging and communicating information on hazards and risks among all concerned parties.

risk management The second step of *risk analysis is the development of policy interventions to control and prevent risk, on the basis of risk assessment and other factors such as their economic, environmental, and social impacts.

risk perception The individual and subjective evaluation of risk as opposed to the scientific and objective evaluation of risk.

saving rate The ratio between savings and disposable income. It can be used as a proxy for the *time discount rate.

selection bias   A bias in the selection process which leads to differentially including or excluding cases with a given characteristic. For example, if one looks at the relation between participation of children in the school breakfast program in different schools and average body weight in these schools, one might find a positive relationship because overweight children are more likely to participate in the program. *See also* Chapter 4.

significance   *See* statistical significance.

social costs   The sum of all *private costs plus external costs (*externalities). In functioning markets, external costs are zero and social costs equal private costs.

social marketing   The application of marketing techniques for social purposes (i.e. to promote a social good); for example, adverts aimed at promoting physical activity.

standards (food standards)   A set of established requirements regulating the characteristics of food products and the production process.

stated preference   Preferences as they are stated directly by respondents through a survey, as opposed to revealed preferences which are elicited indirectly by observing behavior.

statistical significance   A result is said to be statistically significant if it is unlikely that it has occurred owing to sampling error, at a given level of confidence.

technical change   The change in the amount of output produced using the same inputs, thus driven by a change in the production technology.

thin subsidy   A subsidy aimed at promoting consumption of nutritionally healthy goods, as opposed to a *fat tax. *See also* Chapter 4.

time discounting   The empirical fact that economic agents attach a different value to outcomes occurring in different time periods, namely attaching a lower value to outcomes occurring later in time.

time preference   The rate of *time discounting of an economic agent, i.e. the relative preference between immediate and future outcomes. *See also* Chapter 2.

transaction costs   The cost incurred by economic agents to take their market actions. For example, consumers incur transaction costs when they collect and process information to evaluate alternative choices.

treatment group   *See* control group.

underweight   *See* body mass index.

utility   A measure of the satisfaction gained from consumption of a given bundle of goods. *See also* utility function.

utility function   The function relating *utility to consumption levels and to the outcomes of consumption (including health).

value of statistical life   The willingness of society to pay to save one life. For example, if the willingness to pay for a program which avoids 5 deaths out of 10,000 is $1,000 per person, then the value of statistical life is $1,000*10,000/5 =$2,000,000.

waist–hip ratio (WHR)   The ratio of the circumference of the waist to that of the hips.

willingness-to-accept (WTA)   The minimum amount of money that an individual is willing to accept to be deprived of a given good or service (or to be compensated for the lack of policy intervention).

willingness-to-pay (WTP)   The maximum amount of money that an individual is willing to pay to obtain a given good or service (or to benefit from a policy intervention).

Index